The Year I Lay My Head in Water

The Year I Lay My Head in Water

Swimming Scandinavia in Search of a Better Life

Laura Hall

ICON

Published in the UK and USA in 2026 by
Icon Books Ltd, Omnibus Business Centre,
39–41 North Road, London N7 9DP
email: info@iconbooks.com
www.iconbooks.com

ISBN: 978-183773-239-5
ebook: 978-183773-241-8

Typeset by SJmagic DESIGN SERVICES, India

Printed and bound in Great Britain

Appointed GPSR EU Representative: Easy Access System Europe Oü, 16879218
Address: Mustamäe tee 50, 10621, Tallinn, Estonia
Contact Details: gpsr.requests@easproject.com, +358 40 500 3575

For Sarah

I am made and remade continually
Virginia Woolf, *The Waves*

CONTENTS

INTRODUCTION

I was sitting on a bench by Svanemøllen Beach in Copenhagen, scanning passing faces to see if any of them might be a mermaid. Maybe you can spot one if you know what to look out for, I thought. I imagined long hair and a far-away look in pale sea-blue eyes, but perhaps that was just the stuff of stories. A well-coiffed white-haired lady dressed in beige trousers and a light purple jumper threw a ball for her dog on the beach in front of me as I waited. She gave him a snack from a little bag when he came back. Further down the beach, a group of people in dark green waders collected something from the water, perhaps seaweed, in black buckets. A handful of people cycled past along the paved coast path. It was spring but the cyclists were still wrapped in puffa jackets and wreathed in thick scarves. The chilly wind had not yet got the memo that winter was over. I tapped my feet on the floor, trying to get some life back into them as I waited. There was no sign of the lady I had arranged to meet.

My phone pinged. A message from a friend, also a journalist, asking if she could interview me for a story she was writing about mid-life crises. Was I having a mid-life crisis? I wondered. Do people think I'm having a mid-life crisis? I didn't think I was. I felt like I was just dumping all the things I didn't want to do and doing all the things I did. Maybe the mid-life component was that I was old enough to know what these things were, and I was also old enough not to care so much about what other people thought. But then again, what did I know? I was sitting by a beach on an overcast grey morning, clouds heavy with rain above me, waiting for a mermaid. I didn't have anything better to do – and I really mean that, in every sense of the phrase. I didn't have a job, I didn't have anywhere I was supposed to be, and I didn't have anywhere else I wanted to be, either. Even on a cold day, a meeting with a mermaid had a ring of something magnificent to it.

Further down the beach, a pair of Jack Russells were chasing sticks thrown by their owners into the sea, and a woman with long dark hair was balancing something orange-brown and unwieldy on her shoulders beside the snack stand. Something about her hair, whipping in the wind, and the strange shape of the object held my attention. While everyone else was moving purposefully around her, she was standing there, trying not to drop it, but as if she had nowhere else she needed to be either. She was a still point in an otherwise moving scene, and her eyes were fixed on the sea.

Still thinking about my possible mid-life crisis, it took me a minute to realise that the big thing was a tail. And that she was the mermaid I had been waiting for.

I started a swimming journey in Scandinavia at the end of 2019 when I felt burnt out and fed up with life and all of its shackles. I felt strongly, in my bones, that there was a better way to live. If there was anywhere in the world where I could find out how to live better, this felt like it should be the place. Though I couldn't articulate where the idea came from, I felt strongly that I had to find a way to connect with nature more deeply and find something I'd lost along the way. I was looking for a compass to show me where to go, and a spark to set me alive again. At my lowest ebb, I was looking for signs everywhere to point me in a direction that would take me to somewhere better, or just somewhere else. And there was water all around, everywhere I looked.

From where I live in Copenhagen, I see boats sail past my window and the sea shimmer in the daylight that lasts all day long in the summer and passes in a precious flash in the winter. Salt water is the first thing I see in the morning and the last thing I see, as I pull down my blinds, in the evening. It is my view from my desk, my kitchen and my bedroom. I didn't have to go far to find something natural to immerse myself in. I saw neighbours take early morning walks in their dressing gowns down to the deck, shrug off the robes and climb down the ladder to swim, and vigorous and naked twentysomethings take running jumps from the quayside into the harbour while I walked the kids to school. It was all around me, this sign telling me what to do and where to go.

It was a small thing, to start with, dipping a toe into the water just outside my door. But this water flowed into the strait between Denmark and Sweden, to the Baltic Sea that led to Norway, Finland and the Arctic, and to the North Sea that led home to the UK. It was a small thing, but it was part of something much bigger and led, quite naturally, somewhere else.

I started by slipping into the harbour one November morning and it escalated quite dramatically. In a matter of months, I had swum in the Arctic, and by the following September I was swimming in the whale-rich reaches of the Greenland Sea, as icebergs floated past in the distance. I still feel a little baffled thinking about it.

I want to share my swimmer's journey of a year immersed in the cold waters that surround Scandinavia, of the lessons I've learned from swimming with these sea-loving people, Karin the mermaid included, and the perspective it has given me on life. It's a story about what makes you come alive and how doing the things you love can change you in all the best ways. It's about finding a compass that reorientates you to the things that make life worth living. Henry David Thoreau spent a year living in a cottage on Walden Pond to celebrate and honour the value of nature and life itself; I spent my year in salt water.

It all started a few months before I met the mermaid, at the start of autumn.

I. Autumn

1

I felt numb. Nothing seemed [illegible] I did seemed to make any difference [illegible] my job had evolved [illegible] new bosses had come [illegible] new heads of my department [illegible] time, new demands were [illegible] was not keeping up with [illegible] stress to the point [illegible] do anything about [illegible] stress enough that [illegible] was going through the [illegible] sinking to the bottom of [illegible] light glimmering a [illegible] would take a lot of effort [illegible] was easier, always easier [illegible] a little deeper [illegible] I was numb inside [illegible] and I wanted to [illegible] wanted to feel things again.

[illegible] a moment, everything [illegible] happened. I tried to [illegible] but I couldn't [illegible]

1

I felt numb. Nothing seemed to matter and nothing I did seemed to make any difference. It was a work thing: my job had evolved and changed without me realising; new bosses had come and gone with three new heads of my department in the last two years alone, new demands were being made and I was not keeping up with it at all. I was overloaded with stress to the point that I had lost the ability to do anything about it. I stopped caring, and I can't stress enough that that is not like me at all. I was going through the motions. I felt like a stone sinking to the bottom of a pond. I could see the daylight glimmering a bit above me, but I knew it would take a lot of effort to get back to the surface. It was easier, always easier, to let go and stay numb, to sink a little deeper. But I didn't want to feel like that. I was numb inside and starting to go numb all over and I wanted to shock myself back to life. I wanted to feel things again.

For a moment, everything was ice. My lungs tightened. I tried to pull in as much oxygen as I could, but I couldn't get it to go in deep enough.

I panted it into the top of my chest and then out again, shallow as a puddle. The cold burned my skin. There were no thoughts beyond bare survival – in fact, all the racing thoughts that had been filling my time, stopping me from sleeping, making me tetchy, dissolved in an instant. My breaststroke was gaspingly hectic, desperately rapid. It was the panicky stroke of someone new to swimming, afraid of the unknown, someone on the verge of drowning. I was in the ice-cold water for a minute, maybe less, dipped in, holding on to the metal ladder before letting go and swimming for an ice-cold second or two, until I wrestled the tiniest fingertip of control on my breath, calmed down a beat or two, and then I was out, across the wooden decking and wrapped in a towel. My first dip, my first winter swim, was over in a flash. As I exited the water, a bald man in his sixties wearing pink Bermuda shorts executed an energetic dive, entering the freezing cold water headfirst.

It was mid-morning on an early November day in Copenhagen, and all around me students and retirement-aged men and women were dotted along the long wooden quay unwinding their long woolly scarves and folding up their puffer jackets and laughing. The faded sun was shining through the grey sky across the dark water to the city's newest harbour swimming area. Heads bobbed around a section of water the size of a small swimming pool, separated from pleasure boats and ferries by a string of round yellow buoys.

Out of the water, standing on the quay, I was breathing normally again. My skin pinked as I rubbed it roughly with my towel, and then I pulled and dragged my clothes over its still-damp surface. It was too cold to stand in a wet swimming costume for long. I could feel the skin all over my body pulsing. Right through to the end of the day, I had this electrifying sense of my body, and particularly my skin, in a way I had never experienced before. I felt like I was giving off waves of energy.

More than anything else, I felt alive.

If you had told me that day that it would be the start of a year-long cold-water swimming journey across the coldest seas in the world, culminating in becoming one of those people, like the bald Bermudas-wearing man, who dive in off the side of the quay, I would never have believed you. Bruised and burnt out, jobless and hopeless, I was as close to broken as I'd ever been. Days before, I had quit my job with nowhere to go, and nothing but a vague idea that there would be something out there, somewhere. It was a great leap into the unknown not unlike my first plunge into cold water: I didn't know what would happen, or what would come next. I didn't know the water would pull me under, turn me inside out and make me into something new. I just thought that being jobless for a while would be better than the soul-sucking, stress-inducing work that gave me palpitations and such a huge dose of self-doubt that I didn't know who I was anymore.

I wanted to find a way to feel more like myself again. So, I went back to the one place where I felt the most at home.

I was born with a view of the sea from my hospital room, high in Brighton and Hove's tower-block-like hospital to a mum who loved swimming. It was the late 1970s: in the following years, she strolled with her pram and me and my twin brother in it along the promenade past the boarded-up West Pier, which hadn't yet collapsed into the sea. We rolled past the pebbly beaches where family friends had fishing boats resting far beyond the high tide line, leaving traces of tar behind them. Brighton was only a short distance up the coast from where my dad grew up, in Eastbourne, another seaside town we visited regularly, where grand white hotels lined the beach and there was a pier with a shell shop that I saved all my pocket money for. They were quiet seaside towns, back then, alive with holidaymakers in the summer, but out of season, calm, with gardens all the way along the prom styled like thick-pile 1970s carpets. But whatever else there was to do in these towns, all we ever saw was the sea.

Until I was three, I lived a short toddle from Brighton Beach, and I remember swimming in its broth-brown water, and the view of the pier, splashed with cresting waves, as the sun went down and the starlings came in to roost. As I got older, I'd spend summer with my siblings and grandparents by the sea in Eastbourne, poking wine-gum-coloured sea urchins as they clung to the sides of rockpools, followed by Easter on the coast in Suffolk, where my other granny lived and my mum grew up. On this coast, the North Sea, not the Channel, the water was colder, wind-whipped and violent, and swimming was an act of courage. The waves looked like mountains ready to swallow you up. We set up colourful striped windbreaks on the beach, hammering them in with hand-sized round grey stones to cocoon ourselves from the wind, and swam in sea as brown as tea. When the sun came out from behind the clouds, the tiny pieces of sand suspended in the water glittered.

A sports teacher herself, my mum swam in the sea whenever she could, and took us, her children, with her from the very start. A love of swimming was in my blood from the very start, and it only took moving to Denmark, a country where you are never more than 30 miles from the sea at any point, to turn it into a full-blown obsession. From where I sit writing in my apartment in Copenhagen, its sound is always in the air. I've come to know its slack tides and its high spring tides, its occupants and its visitors. I watch it when I can't sleep and it's 3am and the water is so black it looks like oil.

My granny on the North Sea coast swam every week until she was 85 years old, in the swimming pool, in the sea, and wherever she could. She was a champion swimmer in her youth and I owe my love of the water to her utter resilience, to the fact that she unquestioningly swam in water so cold it would make your bones rattle. With a formidable figure like that in your life, it's easy to see where my admiration for swimmers come from. For me, they're the toughest minded, strongest people there are.

My granny taught my mum to swim, just as my mum taught me. I take my daughters swimming whenever I can, here in Denmark, on the other side of the North Sea, eager to pass on my love of the water, an ancestral trait that has a riptide-like pull on the maternal side of the family. Swimming was in my blood, so it makes perfect sense to me that to bring myself back to life, what I needed to do was get back into that cold water and try to start all over again.

2

What took me to the water in Denmark was the exact opposite of swimming. It was a kind of dry drowning. Over the course of a few months, burnout managed to suck me under without me really realising it, like a slow-moving kind of quicksand, or as Hemingway might put it, like bankruptcy. It takes you twice, he says, somehow gradually and suddenly, all at the same time. That's how it was for me with burnout. Something happened between spring and summer that upended my balance without me really noticing. I mean, I was stressed and overworked before then, treating my body like it could work under pressure for a period without breaking, like I was a robot that didn't need rest, continually pushing away the time when I would be able to relax further into the future. Life was like that, sometimes, I rationalised. Except it wasn't just sometimes anymore. By the time the summer holidays were over, I was almost underwater. I had a feeling that if I didn't do something about it, and quickly, I'd drown.

I was working in an office overlooking the harbour in Copenhagen doing a job that I loved. Since my twenties, after training to be a journalist, I'd worked as a travel writer. I'd written stories about travel for magazines and newspapers, I'd written and edited travel guides, mostly about places in northern Europe that I'd always felt inexplicably drawn to, and I'd worked on projects for travel firms around the world. But up to that point in my life, I'd always done it from the UK. I'd always been sitting in England, looking out at the world, spying adventures from there.

When I moved to Denmark, I found a job that fitted me perfectly. It felt like holding gold in my hand, to begin with at least: I was embedded in this part of the world that had captured my interest, and I'd found a way to write about it from the inside. I was part of a team writing about the adventures you could have in this nation, and the playful experiences that encapsulated this part of the world. What started as a fun job became something confusing. Too many meetings, too much work. No chance to catch my breath. Somewhere things went wrong, a connection got lost and I found myself disoriented and dizzy, turned round and directionless. I don't know if I just forgot how many hours there were in the day and overscheduled myself, or if my multiple bosses forgot that I was responsible for a lot of tasks and didn't realise I wouldn't have room for one more, piling more on top of more on top of more. I can't pin down the precise moment that dream job turned into a nightmare, because I was losing track of everything. I got lost in a maze of emails and meetings, each one important, but none of them meaningful in themselves. I was spinning wheels and was unable to get any traction. I was being eaten alive by work.

Although I was working as hard as I've ever worked, I felt like I was going nowhere because much as I was busy, nothing seemed to change. I finished projects and was straight on to the next one, without a chance to review what we'd learned, what we'd noticed, how we'd changed. Things were done, tasks completed, but nothing changed except that I felt depleted with no way to re-energise myself. I've read that burnout can be described as the feeling of coming to the realisation that despite putting your heart and soul into something, nobody else cares about it or you. The idea struck a chord for me. It is painful to give your all and receive just a shrug – if that – for your best efforts. I've also read that burnout is a blocked pathway for stress and that it builds up in your body if you don't find the time for stress relief, for example through exercise. I certainly didn't have that. It can be a feature of people pleasing, of having no boundaries, of taking on too much, of having a poor manager. It is extreme exhaustion in the face of an impossible workload, a growing sense of cynicism, difficulty concentrating, a sense of overall disillusionment. It's a value mismatch between what you're doing and how you feel about the world. It's a weight of expectation that suddenly becomes too much to bear. It's characterised in so many ways and I think I saw myself in just about all of them.

Ding. Another email dropped into my inbox. It was a colleague: are you coming to this meeting? I was late again. Every ding of the email was another drop of water, and the water level was rising. Without me even noticing, it was creeping closer to my chin.

By the time September came around, the water was almost up to my eyes. I was stretching my neck as far as I could, standing on tiptoes to keep my nose and mouth in a position where I could breathe. I was seven years old again and only just able to touch the bottom of the swimming pool. My big toe clawed at the tiles as I tried to keep my footing. It took immense concentration just to stay in this terrifying position, a single step from going under completely.

I left 200 emails unread for months when I came back from a holiday because it felt like there was no way of catching up. There's a horrible sense of loneliness to being in an office surrounded by people but not being able to ask them for help. My friends knew I was having a bad time, but none of them could help, and anyway, they were busy enough themselves. I felt like I'd only take them down with me if I reached out and asked them to help. I skipped lunch with my colleagues and squeezed in a trip to the bakery to eat a white bread roll at my desk alone instead. I asked others in my department and tried to rearrange my workload, but even when projects were reassigned, they somehow still boomeranged back to me with notes saying they weren't quite right, couldn't I just step in and add some ideas? I turned the lights out in the evening as the last person on our floor again, hours after everyone else had left on a Friday afternoon.

At home, my kids were coming home to an empty flat, where their dad cooked dinner just about every night. I fell asleep reading them bedtime stories and sometimes even before. The idea of a social life and friends was a mirage: anyone we did have lunch with at the weekend would meet me as a shell, a half-person, with nothing much to say beyond the fact that work was stressful. Nights were spent staring at the TV from the sofa. My skin was greyish and breaking out all the time and my waistband strained. I was constantly tired but wired. I dreamed about computer screens and meeting rooms, and I woke up with a sore face from grinding my teeth. I'd wake up at 3am nearly every night, thinking about work. It was the last thing on my mind before going to bed, the first thing on a morning. If I just pushed through it, the next phase would be better. I'd be back on top, back in control, once I'd got over this hump.

I carried on, putting pen to paper, typing words after words after words as if they would pull me out of the labyrinth I found myself in. Under the glare of florescent tubes, I wrote about the glories of *friluftsliv*, the Danish love of the outdoors and the general belief that there's no such thing as bad weather if you dress appropriately enough. I wrote about the wide white sand beaches, and the wilds of the northwest coast, where kite surfers carve the air with the edge of their boards. At my corner desk, overlooking a concrete car park, I planned drone videos that swooped and danced along coastlines and through forests, flying up the long lines of clifftop lighthouses and above ink-eyed Jersey cows standing in patchwork fields. I booked into airless, windowless meeting rooms to take conference calls about magical islands and the little ferries that take you to them, and to talk about award-winning restaurants whose chefs forage along the seashore for exquisite-tasting treasures.

Back at my desk, I looked out of the window and thought, *Today's the day I'll get some fresh air. I'll take a walk around the block and clear my head.* But as I stood up to leave, someone grabbed me for a question about another project, and the time dissolved like salt in water.

In the evening, if I could summon the energy to do anything but stare at our TV, it was a miracle. I broke promises to the kids about taking them skateboarding and roller skating, and the dog was lucky if he got to walk beyond a short tour of the block twice a day. I felt broken and guilty, sad for them and sad for myself. So much for *friluftsliv*. In the early autumn, people were still swimming and paddleboarding in the canal outside our house. Meanwhile, our paddleboard gathered dust behind the sofa, unused all year. My memories of enjoying work and life were gathering dust at precisely the same rate. And the irony wasn't lost on me that I was living in Scandinavia, supposedly one of the happiest regions of the world, where work–life balance was cherished. I was definitely doing something wrong.

One Monday morning, the death knell sounded loud enough for even me, with my ears under water, to hear. An envelope was left on my desk with my pay rise information in it. I had a meeting scheduled with my boss – and I was naively hopeful that, since I'd provided information about comparable salaries elsewhere, and all the extra work I'd taken on that year, they'd move me a little closer to the standard rate for this work in the city. I tore it open. Oh.

In that moment I saw a flash of a future where the water rose a half centimetre more, and I drowned. I'd take a month or two off to recover, get signed off sick in the meantime, and I'd dry out. The burnout would lessen and I'd be able to cope again. And then I'd come back to work, grey-faced and changed, forever a tiny bit broken and extra sensitive to stress, to sit in the same seat and do the same thing again, and again, and again, drowning multiple times and taking sick leave every time to compensate until I retired early, my spirit utterly broken. I'd get a pay rise of the same risible amount every year for doing far beyond a reasonable remit of work, and I'd never be valued. I wouldn't be the first.

If existence was about the life in your days, not the days in your life, I was on life support and an alarm was going off in the nurses' room.

I was living a life where I bathed more frequently in fluorescent light than in the harbour or the sea.

I put the envelope, along with its virtually non-existent pay rise, in the bin. I was holding my breath and the water was up to my eyes. I closed them tight, kicked against the bottom and reached up towards the surface. Something in me had snapped and there was no going back. It was time to swim.

I left my job on the last day of October and clung to a flimsy life raft of hope. When people asked me what I was going to do, I cheerfully and opaquely said I was leaving myself open to the winds of fortune and whatever came along. The blitheness hid the truth: I didn't know where I was going or what I was going to do; all I knew was that I needed room to breathe. I tried not to think about how room to breathe has never paid the rent or bought the kids shoes, and even if it ever had done, it wouldn't work in Copenhagen, one of the most expensive cities in the world. I'd have liked a fallow year, a year to do nothing and figure things out, maybe take up watercolour painting or finally join CrossFit, but really, who was I kidding?

In my final days at work, when the unbelievably still never-ending crush of meetings allowed, I daydreamed of what I'd do when I had the space in my day to do what I wanted. What did I want, anyway? I lined up a part time writing job, and left space to think about how to fill in the blanks. I had some savings to tide me over for maybe six months, if I was careful. My husband had a job. Things could be worse, and something would come up. I was willing it to.

I thought about how it felt good to move my body, and how it would really do me some good to do exercise, every day if I could, instead of sitting on a chair in front of a computer all day. This simple and reasonable thing seemed like an almost unreachable dream, and I couldn't quite fathom why. I played sport every day as a student and then life got in the way; although I'd had some obsessive run-ins with the gym in the past, it was no longer a core part of my life. I knew changing that would make me feel good again.

I had started seeing a personal trainer, Christina, once every few weeks in a bid to do something about my weight, but as work had grown to fill more and more of my time, I'd somewhat fallen off the wagon. Blonde and lovely, she was Danish but had lived in Bristol for a number of years, as had I, and it built a bridge between us. I finally didn't feel like a fish out of water in her fitness room. There's something about finding someone who knows the places you know, when you're abroad, and who can laugh at the same things. With children of a similar age too, I felt really understood, perhaps for the first time since I'd moved. Along with her English personal trainer husband, she'd made a life for her family near the beach in the north of Copenhagen and it was a life on their terms. She talked of mornings going horse riding in the nearby ancient woodlands, and of spending long summers in France, reading, researching and planning how to help her groups. She was – is – curious, inspiring, joyful and warm, and I looked forward to our sessions immensely.

I loved her gentle approach – which had taken centimetres off my waist – and the way she greeted me with a pot of freshly made ginger tea before we kicked off each session. I felt we were in it together, and she was just the person I needed to help me get fitter. She knew, way before I realised it, that the weight gain was a symptom and that it was about more than just food. I'd loved seeing her progress in her business, and before long, I thought of her as a friend. I followed her Instagram posts as she put her research and learning into action, eating breakfast outside in the morning to gain a few extra precious rays of sunshine as we moved towards winter, and playing with ideas about what makes a good life, physically and mentally. It was natural that she was the first person I reached out to when things started to come apart at the seams.

I'm on the edge of burnout, I tell her, trying to keep the wobble out of my voice. I hadn't been to see her for a while because I'd been too busy and let things slide. *I'm not over the edge yet but I'm on the brink. What can I do to help manage my stress, and to come out of this period stronger?* In my mind I gave myself a few months to settle into a new way of being and figure things out. It would be fixable, I thought. It wasn't that big of a deal: just a speed-bump in the road, just a stressful period to weather.

Christina's approach boiled down to a few things: mainly focusing on breathwork and treating myself well. Eating healthily, and not skimping on portions, because, as she said, a stressed body craves nutrients. I should get out into green spaces as much as I can, in the middle of the day when the sun is the most powerful, whenever I can. I could feel it already, the slow sink into winter, the grey mornings and the evenings that feel cut off at the knees when you're used the rays of sunshine stretching out to nearly 10pm. In November we consider ourselves lucky if it's still light during a late afternoon commute.

From my desk, I visualised being in green spaces, spending mornings around blue spaces, walking along the beach with the wind in my hair. These are themes I clung to then and thought of again and again when I considered what a good life could be. *If I threw out all the limitations and all the routines that currently bound me,* I thought, *how could life be better?*

I thought back to the things that I had loved as a child. If I wanted to find my spark again, if I wanted to find the real essence of myself, the thing that made me feel alive, it seemed as good as any place to start. Those windswept days on the beach, hollering into the head-high waves, delighting in their cold splash. The goosebumps pimpling grey-pink skin as we came out of the water and dried ourselves off. The brown Thermos flask of tea on Grandma's tartan blanket. The sense of being absolutely, precisely alive in the moment. These were the things to live for, weren't they?

I thought about those people that I saw in the mornings too, the lady next door who swims in the harbour at 6am, and the men who launch themselves naked from the quay just as we're walking around the corner to school. The laughter and the vivid sense of being alive that they embodied.

Christina was the first person I called when I got the idea that I should try out cold-water swimming. There are a few people I'd trust completely with something like this, and she's one of them. I knew she wouldn't laugh, and if something went wrong, she'd know what to do to help. I felt like she'd get why I wanted to do it, and she wouldn't ridicule me for trying. It wasn't something I felt I could do on my own.

For one thing, I was worried about what my body would do. Would I, in the extreme shock of the cold, forget how to swim? Would my heart, given to palpitations anyway, seize up completely? Would I end up in hospital in a gown, its open back displaying my swimsuit? Or would I just slip into the water and never come back up?

I also thought: *What if I don't make a change?* What if cold-water swimming could be a start back to finding my energy again, to feeling like I'm not always pared to the bone or tired to the point that I interpret most things as an insult or criticism, even if that's not what was intended? I just didn't want to be forgetful and confused anymore. I was in no way happy to find myself in this position, but I was glad to feel empowered and confident enough to say that enough was enough. I had just enough energy to steer the ship away from certain disaster. But I didn't really know where I was steering it to.

I was interested in using my own crisis as a springboard to a better way of living, too. From the disarray and rubble of my life, I thought about the castles I wanted to build, and more than that, I thought about how I wanted to feel. I thought about the weightlessness I felt in water, the sleekness and momentum of a glide, the way my fingers cut through the water and the way it bore my weight and helped me move. There was something so natural and powerful about this image in my brain that I felt there was nothing to do but follow it.

3

It was like the beginning of an all-consuming crush: once I'd tried it, I couldn't get the cold water, and how it made me feel, out of my mind. I scoped out a corner of the harbour near my flat, and with my nearly teenage daughter watching on, furtively slipped down the orange ladder and into the dark water. It was a gloomy afternoon and the sun was setting. Clouds were gathering in the sky and a wintry wind was blowing. I knew I shouldn't swim alone, just in case something went wrong. But how wrong could it go, when I was just going to dip in and out, and keep a hand on the metal ladder at all times? Still, I asked my daughter to stand and wait until I was back on land, and told her to run and get help if I looked like I was in trouble.

Sat on the quay watching, my scruffy dog Max barked and strained at the leash, readying himself to jump in and save me, while in the water, my shoulders under its cold shield, I gasped and fought for breath. I tried not to look at the dark green, nearly black water under the wooden platform where the ladder was bolted. Images of black matter, dark green weed, lion's mane jellyfish but black and green in colour, surfaced in my lizard brain. I closed my eyes, willing them away, and focused on my breathing. Then I was out of the water, into my warmest clothes, and home. It was no longer a one-off, but I'll be honest: it wasn't a moment to particularly shout about. It was little more than a dip in the water to remind myself that I was brave enough to do it.

During the previous winter it had been so cold that the sea froze, leaving ducks to waddle about in a bemused way on the ice. I had watched people cut holes in the ice and use metal ladders to dip in and out, and could not imagine why they would do it. I would never have imagined myself doing it. I was afraid of what it would feel like and whether my body was able to handle the shock, and nothing about it screamed fun to me. So it was a kind of a triumph in itself to be swimming on a cold November day, even just for a seconds-long dip. For the rest of the day, I sat bathed in a warm glow at my laptop, and I felt present, again. I could have sworn my skin was still pink – it felt like it should have been a different colour, at the very least. My blood was closer to the surface of my skin than it was before; I became more of a feeling person than a thinking person in those hours after my cold-water shock, and I had a greater sense of my body. After all those months overthinking things, overscheduling my days and forgetting half the things I should be doing, I felt like life had become clear and simple again. It was as if the water had washed the stress clean away, replacing the near-constant panic with a sense of cool control. I was turning up to my part-time job and treading water there while I thought of what the next move would be, when some good fortune came my way. A journalist friend wrote to me with some work: would I take on a feature for him about Copenhagen? It was an obvious yes. It opened a small door for me: I could keep myself afloat by writing about the region where I lived – this time as a freelancer. It felt obvious and a lot less stressful than the way I'd imagined returning to work: if it got too much, I could dip out of it when I needed to. I didn't have to go to meetings. I wouldn't have to work to anyone else's processes. I would only work on things I thought were meaningful. And, as I wasn't chained to anyone's workplace or a 9–5 timeframe, I could go swimming whenever I wanted.

The water itself, flowing outside my door, in and out on the tide every day, was the simple source of it all. Monitored regularly and a source of great pride, Copenhagen harbour has clean waters full of fish, blooming orange jellyfish, and an increasing number of swimmers who take to the waters in floating swimming pools or cordoned-off areas all year round. It's called *vinterbadning* in Danish, or winter bathing, and it's less a trend and more a way of life. It feels like a ridiculous thing to be doing in a European capital city. Of course, Copenhagen is a fraction of the size of London, but just the thought of even paddleboarding on the Thames past important public buildings seems like a kind of madness, let alone swimming past them. I could imagine myself mudlarking along the Thames at low tide in search of old clay pipes from a hundred years ago on a Sunday morning, but I would be afraid that dipping a toe into the water would put me in intensive care. Not so in Copenhagen. Here, as in Denmark and many of Scandinavia's other cities, people regularly enjoy the water, which is crystal clear, and they can swim, paddleboard, kayak and sail all year round. There are fish and thriving marine life under the water, as well as a social life on the top of it and around it. It's all in balance, or just about.

But it's not all plain sailing. The third time I tried winter bathing was definitely not the charm. The wind was raw and it was 8am. I was taking the kids to school and bumped into Mette, another mum from school, who had been swimming in the canals every day for over a year. She invited me along and suddenly I was there, stripped down to my swimsuit, on the platform next to the water. She nimbly climbed in and swam six, seven, eight broad strokes in the shadowy water under her cantilevered flat.

I was trying to persuade my legs to walk down the ladder when she turned and swam back, saying with urgency that she was too cold, she needed to get out. I got thigh-deep in the dark water before I stepped aside and let her get up the ladder. I couldn't get my body to move any deeper. I was too focused on the cold. The fear beat me and I got out.

I felt ashamed. But it was cold, and it was only getting colder. In the next few days, icy weather blew into Denmark and snow began to fall. It was so cold that some days, even with a hat on, I got brain freeze walking down the street to the supermarket. Even though I remembered how great it felt to swim and come out of the water with an electric feeling of warmth around me, I was resigned to not doing it when it was this cold. Maybe in the spring. Maybe when it was warmer. That was it for me.

It would have been the end of my cold-water swimming career if it wasn't for a chance encounter in Norway. An email out of the blue had invited me to write a story for a magazine all about the country's second city, Bergen. It was easily the biggest story I'd snagged so far in my new freelance life, and I was delighted. After a day exploring the city's culture and food scene and an afternoon in the mountains, I found myself with Linn, who works for the tourist board, and an old friend of hers, Stina, for an impromptu swim session by a little pier as the sun was beginning to set. It was about 4pm, just days before the winter solstice when the nights stretch out and steal as much of the day as they can. There were mountains and islands in front of us, little lights glowing in the darkness up the hillsides, and the faint clank of ships' masts and tethered sails against the gentle roar of the waves in the air. Lined up along the quay were a reconstructed Viking boat and pleasure boats waiting for the summer season to return. Linn was first. She swam wide strokes out from the jetty beside the moored boats, and then back. I was next, in the icy water for a few seconds, counting my strokes, breathing wildly, jerkily, before I came out. Then Stina was in, her head right under the water, before she came out again too.

We sat snuggled in blankets in a café afterwards and talked about swimming and how connected it makes you feel with nature. How primal the attraction is. How women have a different relationship with the water than men, and how good it feels to be alive. The picture window of the café framed the sky, sparkling with stars, and the little pier where we'd swam stretched out into the sea. The café was gradually filling up with other winter bathers, who shared their own processes and ideas as they warmed up.

One lady always stayed in the water for as long as she could, more than I could ever imagine, intoxicated by the feeling when her body kicks into gear and starts to warm her up, ten minutes or more after she comes out. Her skin was fish-cold to the touch and she jumped around impishly in the café to warm up. Another, older lady wasn't asking for so much: she just wanted someone to swim with. Pairs of younger women swam and came out, rosy-faced and dripping on to the pier. We sat with our hands wrapped around warm coffee cups talking about swimming and the sea as people came and went and the stars got brighter, until eventually we had to leave.

In that afternoon, the experience became about something more than swimming. It became about what it is to be Scandinavian, what it is to be a woman, what it is to be alive. I felt part of a tribe. If that first rush of endorphins was addictive, this was something else. After four years of living in Denmark, I'd only scratched the surface of what it meant to belong – I'd only really got halfway down the ladder. Now it felt like I was going in deeper.

Inside me, a light was switched on. Inspired by Linn, I resolved to swim in the sea or the harbour once a week, every week, throughout the whole year, to meet other people who swam in the cold seas of Scandinavia, and to see where it would lead. This loose plan glimmered at the edge of my vision: wherever I was, whatever I was doing, I would swim once a week. It was a structure for my structureless days, and I thought that maybe these swimmers held the key to leading a better life.

II. Winter

4

On the last night of the year, I stepped outside at midnight with crowds of others to look at an explosion of colour in the night sky and say goodbye to what had been a difficult year. I wanted to leave it all behind and look to a better kind of future.

The next day, I called my friend Sosun and asked her to swim the harbour with me to see in the new year. I was keen to get my new plan started. Sosun had been swimming since the start of the pandemic as a way to fight stress and had just kept going.

We undressed in the cold air and slipped down the orange ladder, aiming to swim to the second buoy along the rank of parked speedboats in the mini marina facing her flat. Litter from the previous night's fireworks was scattered all along the street and a bottle of Champagne, wrapped in a pink streamer, floated in the green water.

She struck out to the buoy and came back. Then it was my turn. My hangover was coming in waves – nausea, headache, and then it was gone. It was really cold in the water, but my body felt instantly better, tighter, more alive. My head was still woolly: today was not the day to dunk it under.

I've noticed that winter swimmers have rules they set for themselves – maybe they stay in for five seconds, maybe ten. Stina, in Norway, had a rule that she'd always get her head under the water. Linn's rule, which I copied, was to swim every week. Others swim a certain distance, like Sosun, or a certain number of strokes. Perhaps they promise themselves they will dip their head under and they don't feel like they've followed their ritual correctly if they don't. For my part, the intention was just to swim every week for the whole year, a full 52 weeks of swimming. I was not wedded to any particular amount of time but I was aiming to swim at least five strokes before I exited the water. It had to be more than a trip down the ladder and back to qualify.

After climbing out, we sat and chatted on the wooden dock with hands wrapped round rapidly cooling cups of coffee. The endorphin boost from swimming was the absolute best thing about it, but a close second has to be the intimacy and the chat you have afterwards with your fellow swimmers. There's a sense of bonding through having done something daring together that adds heart and soul to an otherwise physical experience. As I was thinking about what life was really for and what makes me really happy, I thought about this too, this sense of community and belonging. How could I find a way to get more of it? How do I fit in, anyway, in a country that I didn't grow up in?

Towards the end of every year, the Danish Language Council, together with P1 radio station, select Denmark's word of the year. In 2020, that word was *samfundssind* – translated as 'community spirit' or 'putting the concern of society higher than one's own interests'. It's the opposite of selfishness, and rang especially true in a year when we had our first lockdowns and the Danish government chose to act first on the interests of the people and second on the interests of business. It's a characteristic I've really noticed in Danish people – a willingness to avoid selfishness as far as possible, whether that's in never taking the last slice of cake in the kitchen at work, in case someone else might want it, or in obeying red lights on empty streets. I remember a lady yelling at me as I casually jumped a red light on my bike in my first year living here. 'Are you so important that you can't wait a minute for it to change?' she asked. She was right. I'm not. Upholding that 'community first' approach is ingrained here, and I was learning it as a foreigner like a toddler on a bike with stabilisers.

It should have been easy to join a community of swimmers, but it is much harder than you'd think. In Denmark, there are more than 93 winter swimming clubs but it's nigh-on impossible to find a space in any of them. As the Danish water safety council noted on its website, the average age for winter bathing used to be 40 but these days it's more like 30 – showing a rising trend among younger people all over the country. *Politiken*, one of the country's national newspapers, even ran a piece called 'What type of Copenhagen swimmer are you?', accompanied by a picture of a naked man, because it was Denmark and nudity is not something that people are shocked by. Until reading it, I hadn't realised there was social climbing involved in swimming, but apparently, depending on where you swim and who you share the sauna afterwards with, you could be looking at better business deals and a tighter, more elevated social circle. The class system seems to be alive and kicking in this otherwise ferociously equality-driven country, in swimming clubs at least.

At this early stage of the game, I wasn't ready to commit to a swimming club, even if there had been a space for me. Waiting lists ran into the hundreds and some clubs near me had closed those lists altogether. I'd have to speak Danish, I expected, if not as a qualification to getting in, at least while I was sitting naked in a sauna next to lots of other Danes. The nudity and the language were both things I struggled a little with and hoped to improve on as time went along. I also felt opposed to paying for something like swimming in the harbour, and having to abide by the laws of the club – swimming has always been about freedom and impulsivity for me. But I did want to find a group I could swim with regularly, for the safety aspect and to help me keep my promise to myself – to just keep swimming, week by week.

Even though the last year felt hard, spirit-crushing and demoralising, in just a few months, the experience had given me something great. I reached a turning point where I could ask myself: what do you want? What makes you happy?

Now, nearly every day, the answer was simple: 'swimming', on my own, with a friend, in the harbour, in the sea. It was just swimming.

Something had happened to life after the pandemic lockdowns that made its edges blunter. The idea of risk, now we had come face to face with it all over the world, had become too dangerous, too real. So life, for me, for many of us had become a cocoon. We stayed home instead of going out, muffled from the world.

Snow fell outside but we didn't rush out to see it or feel it kiss our eyelashes. I felt a sense of daring ebb away in me, courage leaking tiny drop by tiny drop, until taking a bus into town seemed like a challenge, let alone taking on the world. We stayed in, watched Netflix, waited to be told what to watch next. Algorithms on social media and through our technology took decisions for us, until making one ourselves, using independent thought, felt risky.

It becomes hard to practise courage when you're spending a lot of time in your own cosy surroundings on the sofa. It takes courage to do so many of the things we had all collectively done over those years – facing up to a fear of needles, working in the healthcare service or in a shop – and while a lot of people had been practising it, I was one of the army of people that hadn't been very courageous. I'd lived a little life, a smaller life, in those few years, and a less ballsy one.

Curled up on my pink sofa, I read and read. In Brené Brown's *Dare to Lead*, she says that we are starving for opportunities to be courageous. She talks about how courage is a muscle that you can flex, and the more you do it, the stronger the muscle gets. It's a behaviour, not a character trait. I knew I could do with more of it.

Swimming in the cold harbour became my act of weekly bravery. I was never quite sure if I'd really do it until I did. I nearly bottled it every time my feet reached the water. Keeping going was a core part of it all. Just like being brave is not about being unafraid, it's about being afraid but doing it anyway, swimming in cold water isn't about the swimming, it's about facing up to how cold or uncomfortable it will be and still doing it, even though the water will chill you to the bone. Sometimes it was because I wanted to feel something, but often it was because I needed to prove to myself that I still could.

In a very small part of me, it was like a light had been switched on. I felt a little bigger than I was and a little more confident. At work, where I was floating about as a freelance writer, when I took the initiative to meet new people and to approach potential clients about work, I could feel that my tone had changed. I was making progress in terms of my confidence and attitude.

There were other areas of my life where a newfound sense of bravery could really have an impact. Speaking Danish was one of the obvious ones. I'd had lessons but it's a tricky language and nothing seemed to stick. I made so many mistakes and mangled so many words that I felt self-conscious about it all. There's nothing like being laughed at when trying to speak a language for making you feel like you'll never try again. I wanted to get better at it. But could I be courageous enough? Maybe the swimming would help.

5

I was not the only one new to swimming in Copenhagen harbour. A seal arrived in the south part of the harbour one winter night, a chubby little silver-grey lump beached on a platform usually reserved for kayakers or fishermen beside a bridge leading to the open sea. I took my youngest daughter on a moonlit walk to find it, when she'd normally be brushing her teeth and getting ready for bed. There were a few people standing on the bridge in the dark, just looking at it: its pelt glowed in the bright white streetlights. It didn't look at all concerned by the gawpers on the bridge, or the roar of the traffic from the nearby motorway. It lay like a sunbather on a beach. We stood in the dark, fingers and toes getting numb, looking at it roll and twitch, until we couldn't take the cold any longer, and headed home for hot chocolate.

We went back a few days later and were disappointed that it wasn't there. We leaned on the railings and talked about how it's not a good thing to touch it, if it ever came close enough, because mother seals can reject their babies if they smell humans on them. Sometimes stepping in to save something can be an act of vandalism that puts happiness out of their reach. It felt profound, standing in the wind, to think that it was better for them to help themselves and learn in their own way to thrive, than to step in and help. Then, with a squeal of joy, someone pointed from the bridge. A little round wet head with liquid eyes broke the surface of the water, bobbed about for a moment, then returned to the shiny school of mackerel it was chasing.

Denmark's wildlife rescue service, *Dyrenes Beskyttelse*, said that it's not that uncommon to find seals in the harbour. Apparently, there are a lot of them about, especially in winter, when there are plenty of fish in the harbour and plenty of young hungry seals ready to eat them. It seemed likely that the fish drew the young seal in, and that it wasn't lost, or ill. It just needed a safe and easy place to learn to catch fish and fend for himself.

We changed our usual dog-walk route to go past this part of the neighbourhood once a day, just to check in on him. It made the front page of our local area's newspaper. I was happy to swim in a harbour that was clean enough to attract a wild seal. But it did raise a shadowy thought about how deep the harbour was, how big the fish at the bottom were, and what lay beneath. I didn't want to think about these things. All of us swimmers lock away that thought so it doesn't surface and stop us from doing what we love. The area where the seal hunted was, anyway, some distance from where I swam, almost a whole island away.

At least that's what I thought, until a photo on our neighbourhood Facebook group showed a paddleboarder being closely investigated by the seal. In the selfie, the paddleboarder stands on a pink and white inflatable board, paddle in hand, while over her shoulder, the seal is almost mouthing the back end of the board, like a puppy testing its teeth. The buildings in the background gave away the location – and to reach it, the seal must have swum right past Sosun's house, and the marina area where we sometimes swim.

What would it be like to swim with a seal? I was afraid it might be territorial like a dog, and could nip or bite. Our local seal might be small but that didn't mean anything. I'd spent enough time watching them in the zoo, swimming as fast as a missile when they wanted to, even after years of being in captivity. Splattered with light grey spots and nearly as long as one of my legs from nose to tip, our seal might have been as cuddly as a pillow and as curious as a puppy, but I'd be careful next time I was in the water.

It reminded me, for a moment, of when I lived in Bristol, a harbourside city that feels like a cousin to Copenhagen. Its old docks are alive with life again too, and multicoloured houses also line its old seafaring waterways. The only time I remember anyone going swimming in the brown, silty Avon, though, was when they got too drunk and fell off the quay in the summer. One winter there was a rumour that there was a crocodile in the harbour and we rushed to see if we could find it, not because we really thought we'd see one, but because, this being creative, beautiful, ebullient Bristol, it could have been an anarchist stunt, or a pop-up artistic statement, or something even more delightfully odd and unexpected.

A real seal, though, seen with your own eyes. That was something else.

In the dark winter nights, I read *Letters from Tove*, a sprawling book collecting together Tove Jansson's personal letters, gifted to me by a friend in Finland. The Finnish author, known globally for her white hippo-like Moomins, had enjoyed the most enviable life as a young woman, taking avant garde art classes in her early twenties in Paris, travelling at will throughout Europe, and working on her art, writing and ideas as she went, as a vagabond bohemian artist who found her food everywhere. Reading about her life in the 1930s, jealousy nipped at me gently. To be with this crowd of creative people, to be this talented … it seemed like my idea of a wonderful life. I noticed the envy: it wasn't an emotion I felt ashamed of, but one I knew I should take note of. *If I'm feeling jealous,* I thought, *maybe it's a signpost on the way to the life I want to live.* I noticed that Tove didn't spend her days writing in a concrete box of an office, rather on a deserted rocky island with seagulls and waves for company, along with a sauna in the basement. A girl can dream.

After a decade of having small children at home, with the tight weave of schedules and the weight of responsibility that they bring, my life reckoning was coming at a time when the future looked freer than it had for years, though hardly on a par with Tove Jansson's. The unchartered territory before me was dazzling. Witnessing how else life could be lived set a fire in me. Now that I was freelance, unshackled, I didn't have to play by the same rules as everyone else. The kids still needed me, of course, but the weave had loosened as the years went on and they had become much more independent, and even more so now we were getting more settled in Danish life. In true Danish style, in year three (age nine) my eldest was instructed to walk to school alone and pack her own school bag; she now went to and from school alone, often picking up her younger sister in the afternoon too. The lack of mental stress, the lack of constant timekeeping that had dogged my days at the office, hurrying from meeting to meeting, being pulled in every direction, offered up a blank canvas to paint on. Perhaps I could set the rules of my own life?

I kept to my timetable of swimming at least once a week, and as I did, I saw something interesting in the women I swam with, and the women I saw at the beach in these raw days of winter. Sometimes there were a gaggle of younger girls together, shrieking and laughing, enjoying the dare and thrill of the cold water. But more often, more visible to me, anyway, were the older women, the ones aged forty and up, who swam quietly in twos and threes, wearing black costumes and a colourful woolly hat, the unofficial costume of the winter bather.

They were friendly, usually, but not overly so. Like all Danes, they seemed to believe that it's good to give each other space – something I've seen described as a negative, but which is really a positive. They wouldn't speak to you unless you asked for help, and then would be more than happy to pitch in. Otherwise they assumed that everything was fine. It's all about preserving your privacy and dignity, giving you the gift of personal space.

Were they like me? I wondered. Maybe they were escaping the constriction of family life too, and were shunning the rigidity of the modern workplace. Maybe it was the menopause. Maybe they were looking for challenge and excitement in unlikely places and it was better than having an affair. I wondered, not for the first time, about why there were so many women swimming in the cold sea, and not so many men. Why us, why now?

It was a curious thought that I would come back to again and again over the year. It was a comfort too, to feel that I fitted into a tribe already, even if I was only on the fringes of it.

In mid-January, I took a trip to the seaside with Effi, a friend who wanted to try winter bathing for the first time. January feels like an open door to push when it comes to new things. It was a new year, why not try winter bathing? Why not ride a scooter for the first time? Why not shoot for the moon if you want to? She was more up for it than anyone I'd seen, embracing January with a full list of 31 brand new things to do to mark the new year, and swimming in the winter sea was right at the top of it. With the blank page of the new year ahead, everything seemed possible. I suggested a place I've always wanted to swim: Kastrup Sea Bath.

This beautiful seawater bath is perched off the beach in Amager Strand, an artificial beach near the airport in Copenhagen. On a good day, you can sit on the beach and see planes circling and coming into land, while also looking across the sea to Sweden. The Turning Torso Tower in Malmö is a landmark I always look for, a twisting column standing tall in the distance like a tower built of white Lego blocks. Bright-painted cargo ships passed in-between us on a trade route to the Baltic Sea from Germany and beyond. By January standards, the weather was fantastic – the temperature was due to range from 3 to 6°C, admittedly very cold, but the sky was the false blue of a summer's day, that blue that makes everything feel possible. Walking along the beachfront trails were people fully wrapped up in scarves, gloves and coats, topped with sunglasses.

I had been thinking about swimming all week. While everything else had been wheeling in a hectic way around me, it was a still point I was looking forward to.

Kastrup Sea Bath is a conch-shape, a circular structure with a wall winding from low to high around it to protect swimmers from the wind. Inside the wall, there are benches and spaces to get changed, platforms to jump from and ladders for the more cautious. Lights embedded in the wooden walkway show the way to the water in the darker months. It's set out to sea along a pier, so you don't have to wade through the shallows to get deep enough to swim. Swimming piers are a common feature along the gently shelving Danish coastline for this reason – it takes a while to get deep enough to swim, and while Danes are a patient people, they are also very good at designing around problems and finding neat solutions. This way, you can be in the water quickly with no wasted time. When you want to swim, you can swim.

It's called the Kastrup Sea Bath but locals call it the *snegl* – a word that simultaneously means 'snail' and a type of pastry that has a snail-like whorl shape. The sky sat heavy on our shoulders, but the water, lapping gently at the platform, was translucent and light turquoise-blue. Underneath it, dark brown seaweed drifted over the pale sand.

This being Denmark, the first thing that greeted us was a naked man of a certain age, who pranced around the platform limbering up before plunging in and swimming broad, wide breaststrokes as if it was a warm summer's day and nobody was watching. He made a great show of swimming before he got out and cavorted around a bit more to dry himself off. We gave a collective sigh of relief when he left, and only women remained at the swimming spot, in clumps of twos and threes.

Two women I judged to be over 50, maybe 60, swam directly across from us in bright woolly hats and black swimsuits, with black neoprene socks on their feet. They plunged their shoulders under the water, laughing and counting at the same time before exiting the water. After warming up, they did it again, chatting all the while as if they were at a knit and natter session in a cosy café.

I stripped off quickly, and walked down the wide plank steps, noting the floating seaweed fronds as I got further in. It was entirely different from swimming in the closed water channels in the harbour – the sea felt freer, cleaner, clearer and, despite the wooden enclosure, more open to the world.

I swam a few strokes, breathing deeply, and felt good. I could feel the progress – although my breath caught immediately and my lungs constricted, I was no longer as shocked by the cold, and I recovered quicker, able to swim more freely and even breathe properly while I was in there. I counted five broad breaststrokes and then I climbed out. Out of the water, my feet didn't feel so icy. Maybe it was just that it was now warmer, and the sea was warmer than the harbour. Maybe it was because – in another sign of growth – I'd brought an extra towel to stand on so my feet would warm up quicker.

I filmed Effi on her phone – proof is always needed of these big events – as she stepped into the cold water, put her shoulders under, and came out. She chatted nervously, trying not to show she was scared. But she was scared, just like I had been: scared of what her body might do, unsure of whether she would have a panic attack or a heart attack, and whether she could stand the cold or not. She was all smiles when she came out, relaxed, and even, ten minutes later, regretting not staying in for longer. It's a great relief to know you can trust your body not to have a meltdown. Even better to see someone else go through it and realise that they are stronger than they thought they were. We'll go again, we promised when I dropped her off. How about February?

It was rewarding to induct someone else into this mad pursuit. I mean, it was me, concerned about my freezing feet, worried I might bottle it, just a few months ago. Now I was the one sharing my second towel and encouraging someone else to breathe. As we walked back across the bridge to the shore, a dark cormorant bobbed to the surface with a live crab in its beak. The crab's legs clawed at the air until it, along with a long strand of emerald-green seaweed, was swallowed whole and the beady eyes of the cormorant spied something else to eat.

It reminded me of that mantra 'eat the frog' – the idea that you should do the big, hard things first, and then everything gets easy from then on. The cormorant ducked down under the water and disappeared, in search of its next snack, no doubt. It reminded me that I'd done the hardest thing already: I'd looked my life in the face and said it wasn't working. I'd quit my job and found a way to work that was helping me get better. And I was at the beginning of a journey to figure out what a better life might be.

6

When you live in a harbourside community, the sound of water becomes the subtle soundtrack to your day. Twice an hour, the harbour bus, our local public ferry, made its slow chug up the water and down to the tighter channels and canals, stopping outside our flat for ten long, thrumming minutes before moving on. In the summer, the squeals and splashes of people jumping in from the deck outside our flat brought some fun into the heavy air. In the winter, when it was really cold, it made a different sound, slower and thicker, somehow. Scientists have found that salt water is denser and more viscous when it's cold, so that makes sense. It was so cold at the end of January that when I walked the dog in the early evening under a black sky, the water gathering in the corners of the canals slushed together, thickening. Last year the canals froze completely and houseboats were locked in the ice.

On a late January day, the sun was glittering on the water from halfway up in the perfect blue sky and something wonderful happened. There's a lovely word in Swedish, *mångata*, which we'd translate more prosaically to moonbeam, but which in Swedish means a path lit by the moon, a moon road or moon street. That's how the sun looked, shining in a clear broad line on the water, calling me in. A *sungata*.

I took the dog for a walk and felt the sun on my face, the wind gentle for the first time in days, past Sosun's flat. I've started to call round at hers in the way I used to call at my friends' houses when I was little, only instead of asking if she can come and play, I ask if she wants to swim. She was at the window but couldn't be persuaded – it was a Friday lunchtime and she had a series of online meetings ahead. I shrugged. Maybe I'd go by myself anyway. I didn't really want to swim alone – it felt risky, and thinner, somehow, than doing it with someone else. But the sun was stronger than it had been for months, and the water was calling.

Before I entered the water, two women wrapped in winter coats with woolly hats on stopped to chat. I'd seen one of them before – her children went to the same school.

'You're brave,' one of them said. I was standing on the wooden pier in my swimming costume and a salmon pink hat.

'What makes you say that?' I said.

'Swimming on your own,' she said. 'I have to have a deal with my friend,' she nudged her, 'otherwise I wouldn't do it!'

They said they swam every morning after the school run. I told them I would love to have more people to swim with, I was only doing it on my own out of necessity, and maybe after the school run could work for me, too. We swapped numbers and arranged to swim together the following week.

When they had gone, I stayed under for the longest time yet, luxuriating in the emerald-green water. I didn't even count the strokes – I'd stopped feeling that I had to force myself to stay in for longer than I could bear. I could bear it. I could bear it for as long as I wanted. I breathed in deeply and noticed my legs and my feet as they soaked in the cold of the water. It slowly crept up from my toes to my calves. I climbed up the ladder and got out.

It was a new swimming spot for me, a right turn along the harbour instead of a left at a pier nestled between a marina of small boats. I sat in my swimsuit, wrapped in a navy-blue towelling dressing gown, for a while, thinking about how great and necessary it was to meet some more swimmers. The air was the warmest it had been for weeks, around 4°C, and I sat on the wooden bench as the saltwater soaked into my robe. It felt like I'd undergone a transformation.

When I got home, there was a text on my phone:

> Hi Laura, Nice finding a winter mermaid. Let's find a spot for next week to swim.

It buoyed me up, a little air bubble pulling me up to the surface. It might be one of the best texts I'd ever received. I'd been starting to think about how

I could find a regular group to swim with and it just appeared.

I'd been wanting to meet some new people since leaving my job and working mostly alone at home. When I've been at my lowest ebb, meeting new people has been really challenging. But as I started to pull away from the depths of my burnout and hopelessness, I noticed that I wanted to. As well as giving me a tiny framework to wrap around my otherwise unstructured days – one dip a week as a minimum – I started to think that swimming was about being part of something bigger than myself. It was about being part of the world around me, the world outside my flat. It made sense that as well as joining the natural world and temporarily becoming part of it, I'd start to rejoin a social world that I'd been absent from for some time. The confidence boost I was getting from it, the energetic, slightly hyper feel I would have when I got out of the water, propelled me forward. Back to that 'eat the frog' idea: when you've done something challenging, other things feel easier by comparison.

I started to think about how I could make stronger links with Danes, given that most of my friends were expats of some description, and most of my Danish friends were ex-work colleagues. At the same time, I was thinking about how life is richer lived with friends of different ages, and how, without my extended family nearby, I didn't see as much of older women as I had in the past. Almost certainly, it's because I was terrified of speaking awful Danish to older people – for some reason I had got it in my head that they would be more unforgiving of it. But I came to realise that if I never did it, I would never do it. And that's how I found myself on the edge of the harbour at seven o'clock one freezing January morning with two older women, naked apart from their bobble hats.

Jette was the boss of a friend of mine and I had heard she liked winter bathing; Hanne was a textile artist, and both of them were kind enough to let me join them on their daily swim. I hadn't been up and out of the house this early for years. It was still over an hour until sunrise, and my teeth were chattering.

Jette and Hanne were warm and effusive, happy to share details about swimming as we walked along the moonlit cobbles to the edge of the water. There are just two things you need, explained Jette. An S-hook so you can hang your handbag above the wet floor. The deck we were standing on was still wet from the previous days' snow. And you also need a second towel to put on the ground for when you get changed and when you come out, so your feet don't freeze.

We'll keep our hats on today, said Hanne. She then stripped off completely and jumped in. Jette did the same. I was momentarily dumbfounded – I thought our mutual friend Cecilie's message last night that 'real winter swimmers do it naked' was a joke. It wasn't. These ladies were the real deal. I stripped off as quickly as I could down to the swimsuit I had on underneath my clothes, and followed them in.

The lights shone in the black harbour as waves formed and bulged, pushed along by the commuter-hour harbour bus, and we all swam in the cold water for a few brief moments before climbing out. Swimming in inky darkness before sunrise had a deep sense of mystery to it. Though I didn't put my head under water, the stress headache that had been forming ahead of a day of meetings had gone completely.

As we towelled off, we talked about the energy boost that swimming can give you, and the stress relief it creates. Hanne said she started swimming because she got migraines and she thought it would help. Jette said simply that it was the best way to start the day, every day. Even on a cold black morning in winter. I can see why: beginning the day with something that reaffirms to yourself how brave you are, and jolts your endorphins into action, is definitely a good thing. Though it's cold and dark outside, inside I feel full of energy.

The sun was starting to fray the dark edges of the sky as I waved goodbye to them and cycled off to my meetings. 'Come any time – we meet at 7.15am every day,' they called after me. Maybe next time I'd be brave enough to swim naked too. From swimming almost secretively on my own to joining a nascent swimming group and dipping with some Danes, things had really turned a corner.

7

One Sunday morning, hours after a storm ravaged Copenhagen and raised the water level in the harbour by two metres, my friend Sunčica and I went on a Viking raid. There was already drama in the air, and litter whirling in the wind and down the street, as we approached the National Museum of Denmark. Inside, a new exhibition was bringing to life a vivid period of Scandinavian history: the time of the Viking raids. We were to join chieftain Bjørn Ironside on an interactive expedition across place and time.

The exhibition was in the main hall, heralded by a flag of a dead warrior laid on autumn leaves, sword in the centre of his chest, weeping wife at his side. Inside, thousand-year-old gold rings and pendants studded with precious stones glittered in glass cases like gems in a fine jeweller. We picked out our favourites, noses pressed to the glass, like teenagers planning a fantasy wedding.

Seeing Viking history in a Danish museum as an English person is like looking at history through the opposite end of a telescope. I felt like a spy behind enemy lines: seeing the English from a Viking point of view brought up some interesting thoughts about the people I lived among every day.

The Vikings have always been my favourite part of history. I can remember standing in the ruins of Lindisfarne Priory as a child, looking out across the North Sea, imagining striped sails appearing on the horizon. It was a day when it rained and rained and we mistimed the tidal crossing and were forced to hole up in a pub for hours, just my mum, my toddler sister, spotted with chicken pox, and me. But it was worth it for that fervour, that gold-lust. *The Vikings are coming*. The thump of my heart.

As an adult, I think I should have felt the blood run cold in my veins, not this prickle of excitement. The Vikings were, let's remember, a tribe of warriors who set fire to our villages, pillaged our churches and took our women and men as slaves. It ought, perhaps, to make us feel ashamed, vulnerable and colonised. Maybe we should feel smaller, less than these Danes who barrelled in and occupied more than half the country from East Anglia through to the border with Scotland and much of the Midlands for nearly 200 years. We should fear them, not revere them. They should be the enemy.

A small part of me wonders, though, if after so many years of being ruled by them and integrating with them, we are them. Danish blood runs through all the parts of the north of England where I grew up, and where my parents live now in Cumbria names like Motherby, Shap, Lazonby and Langwathby bear echoes of their Danish owners. Perhaps the blood thumping in my veins is Danish after all.

It's also human nature to admire the fire in their eyes, their drive to conquer the world, take whatever they like and be bound to no rules but the ones they want to set. It's a kind of wish fulfilment. Sitting on hard plastic seats in an itchy school uniform, it's no wonder English school children like me were captivated by stories about a tribe that seemed to make its own rules and never curb its appetites an inch.

In the museum, a handful of panels explore the story of the Vikings in England, from the raids on Lindisfarne to their subsequent occupation of the north of England and the reign of King Canute. This is our story of the Vikings, the story I read growing up in England, and part of the patchwork of stories I studied as an undergraduate at Oxford, steeped in Anglo Saxon and Old English. As a nation, England experienced this brutality, and the subsequent rule of the Danes over half of the country, but as part of Denmark's national history, it is only a slice of the broader story of the Scandinavian tribes that traversed the globe, settling Iceland, reaching Newfoundland, and voyaging as far as Russia and Egypt.

In one of the explanatory videos, a curator talked about how the Vikings came in waves to England, first to steal, and then to settle, bringing their families in longships over the North Sea to found farms. 'The dream of improving one's life by migrating is one we have always had,' she said. It seemed like she was just talking to me.

Instead of moving west, my family and I went east, and a thousand years behind schedule, but we were in search of a better life all the same. In place of the Viking need for fertile ground for our livestock and vegetables, we came for a more balanced work–life balance and a focus on a sustainable future. You can't measure it in gold, and it would make a pretty mundane TV show, but they are modern-day riches all the same. Why, despite this set up, there are so many people that I have worked with or know well who suffer from burnout is another question I can't easily answer. Perhaps it's just that some things are better and some things are worse, and you won't know until you get there. Or perhaps we've all lost our way and misread our compasses just a little, even those of us in Scandinavia. Perhaps we should all go back to the water and what it can bring us.

Beyond the glittering treasure cases, the exhibition led on to an interactive journey where we would travel with Bjørn Ironside in search of the legendary city of Rome. We suffered alongside the Vikings as they rowed with salty hands and camped on boggy ground. Besieged near the rocks of Gibraltar, blazing arrows struck our ships, our sails caught light and we died in a rain of fire. Our dead bodies sank like lead weights in the sea, falling, falling through an ombre of sea-glass green to black for the goddess Rán to claim.

According to legend, Rán was the maker of all the storms in the northern oceans. She dragged people down to the depths of the ocean with her net and collected their souls. She was tragically beautiful, with blue-green skin and long black hair that trailed away into seaweed.

She was a goddess you would trust your treasures to, sinking them in a bog with reverential words before you journeyed, and a goddess that mothers would curse when the ships bearing their sons never returned. She was a widowmaker and a treasure keeper and she was the dark side of the sea. I had a daydream about what it would have been like back then, to wave the men in your life off to sea, not knowing if you'd see them again. To offer everything you had to the sacrificial pond, pieces of silver, gold and pottery, to beg the gods to bring them back safely. And then to stand in the sea, fighting it, cursing it, with saltwater tears streaming down your face when you discovered that Rán had decided to make you a widow and take them for herself anyway.

Outside the museum, the wind had eased off a little but still howled and pushed us down the street all the same. The water was still racing in the harbour, a day after the storm. It didn't feel like the same water I had swum in a few days before, back when the wind was resting and the sky was blue. The Viking goddess of the sea was reminding me not to get complacent about the power of the elements.

On the bus back to my flat, I browsed a Sunday newspaper and started reading a story about micro-management and the toxic workplace. My heart started pounding. I couldn't make it to the end of the article, stopping at a passage where an employee says she staggered her working day to avoid a particular character who made her life hell. It sounded a bit too familiar. I was instantly transported back a few months to disagreements at work, difficult colleagues and a sense of helplessness about how to handle all of it. The feelings of being overwhelmed and overworked flooded over me again. I'd been complacent about getting over burnout. Just because I wasn't in the same workplace anymore, it didn't mean I had escaped it, or even healed yet. It had only been a few months. These things can still rear up out of seemingly nowhere.

Like Rán lurking in the depths, that sense of burnout and hopelessness was still there, just under the surface. Like the sailors of the past, I needed to be careful, to be prepared and thoughtful. I needed to keep tight control over what I took on and what I prioritised. Otherwise, maybe I too would go under.

8

It wasn't long before I started feeling like things were falling apart again. I always catch the blues in February, in that dark month where all progress seems to stall. I was feeling listless, unmotivated. Unclear about the future and with a gnawing feeling in my belly that I'd made a huge mistake. The confidence that weeks before had been blossoming, had now receded. Now that this decision to leave the classic world of work had been made, and the novelty had worn off, it all looked a bit different. It looked foolish, really. It looked like I'd risked it all. Perhaps all I had needed was some time away from the office, I bargained with myself. Perhaps I had needed a rest. And now, more back to myself again, I needed to go back to work.

Much as artificial light and office life felt so wrong to me, I was doubting my decision to leave them behind. I felt invisible, still jobless and aimless. Being freelance was all very well, but it was hardly secure and it felt so unsteady. I was not even sure what I wanted, let alone how I was going to find it. So much for the good life, and finding a better way to live it.

I started helping another company with their website content, in a bid to feel connected to the world of work again, like an adult. I left in the dark morning and the sun had sunk well before I got home. But far from buoying me up, the return to office work sunk my mood as well. It seemed I couldn't win.

Seasonal malaise wasn't a new thing for me, but moving to Scandinavia hadn't helped. I guess that nobody is truly happy during a long, dark, wet winter, even if they do have the right clothing and have grown up with it. Without a car, there was no insulation from the months of grey skies and the seemingly never-ending blustery cold.

The only thing I could do was keep the promise I'd made to myself to keep swimming once a week and try to see that as a way forward. As I looked through climate data, I saw that February was the month with the coldest seawater in Copenhagen, with an average sea temperature of 2.3°C. The weather website that I browsed had this information too:

> *Note: For swimming, this is considered life-threatening and very dangerous. The water feels painfully cold, and hyperventilation quickly occurs. A specialized swimsuit is mandatory to reduce thermal damage.*

A specialised swimsuit? Uh, maybe not. I just swim in my regular swimsuit these days, just like the others I swim with – except for the ladies who swim nude, that is.

I tried to fight off the blues with a SAD light, supposed to help with seasonal affective disorder, and I knew I should step out into the light at lunchtime whenever I could, just to get a little Vitamin D into my body. I took supplements by the handful too. But the truth was, it was not just the weather that was getting me down. I was overwhelmed at work again, taking on too many projects, not having a clear enough view on how long it would take me to do things and how much I could do. I'm a *tidsoptimist* – a delightful Danish word meaning I'm over optimistic about how long it takes me to do things, assuming everything will take less time than it does – and I found myself more stressed than I'd have liked to be as a result. It felt like that familiar sinking feeling from a few months before.

A Danish saying goes that 'it is too late to learn to swim when the water is up to your lips'. It seemed to fit. I took some time to think about what I was doing, and why I was saying yes to everything all over again. I think it was just that saying no is hard when you are living week to week. It's hard when the projects coming your way look like fun. I hadn't expected to be in this position.

I spent some time with some businesswomen that I knew and used them as agony aunts. 'How do I stop myself getting burnt out again?' I asked. And then more specifically, but related: how do I manage this unmanageable workflow where I don't know what's coming around the corner?

The answer to the first question could apply to a lot of things, but that didn't mean it wasn't true. Getting over an emotional event is not a linear process. There will be stumbles and missteps. You may have to step backwards before you can leap forwards. The sooner you realise this, and cut yourself some slack, the sooner things will move forward. You can't fight the process, and everyone gets through it at a different pace. So it's just about time, being kind to yourself, noticing your triggers and pulling back when things are too much. Stopping short of burnout this time meant doing things differently from last time, and slower and more intentionally, if possible. I reminded myself of another mantra I had found useful in the past: there's no rush. Life is long as well as short. Thinking about a longer horizon than right now always has a way of making me feel calmer.

For the second, there was an easier answer: I just had to learn to say no. It doesn't have to be said in the moment – one friend advised me to take longer to make decisions, to say that I'd get back to people, or to leave off replying to emails for a day, to give me more thinking time. I resolved to try.

My head was still buzzing with thoughts about how everything felt wrong when I met up again with my new winter mermaid friends Hanna and Sonia. We met at the deck near my house, a square of wooden planks attached by a little bridge to a cobbled footpath that ran beside the harbour. The wind whistled past it, and buffeted the small boats docked along the marina nearby, giving off strange clanking sounds. In the winter, it was deserted and dusted with snow, but come summer, the deck here would be packed with people like hot dogs on a grill, glistening with sun cream.

It was cold underfoot. We left our bags and towels on the picnic tables, and Hanna hung her towelling gown on the wall by the ladder. I was keen to get in but hesitated. I stood in my swimsuit in the wind chatting while the others changed, unwinding long wool scarves and discarding multiple layers. I was waiting for one of them to go in first. I felt like I was rushing them.

Then we were in, rinsed in ice-cold water all over our bodies from our shoulders to our toes and the tips of our fingers. The cold was a pause, a moment out of the world, where all there was to think about was swimming and no stress or worry beyond that existed. Then out, into towels, then semi-dry and back into clothes. Sonia was buzzing with energy when she came out, ready to take on the world. I was not, but that was OK. My body was cold to the core, but finally my head was calm. My jittering thoughts had found some peace; all the negative self-talk about how bad I was at building the perfect life for myself stopped for that moment. Being cold was as good as a slap in the face for my spiralling thoughts.

The bad February experience in general made me think. I hadn't really done anything about my feeling of burnout except change jobs and hope it would go away. Without any preparation of how to approach it, my negative thoughts were going to overwhelm me every time I came across anything a little stressful, I could see that. I needed to start being aware of the signs that those moments were coming, and find techniques to help me ride them without being pulled under.

I started to build a plan of how things could look three, six and nine months ahead, and how I could anticipate, spot and nix any problems before they became too deep. I dreamed too, surfing travel websites and Instagram for new places to go, and stumbled on a heated pool in Helsinki harbour that looked like heaven. A more defined plan emerged beyond my once-a-week swimming programme. What if I can take it further and swim more? Maybe I should take a Scandinavian tour of some of the best and wildest places to swim? Taking on this seascape of adventurers and mermaids, looking at how and why other people swam, and joining them to see if it changed my view of the world felt exciting. I suddenly had a plan.

9

Scandinavian travel was on the agenda, but not quite how I had imagined. In the middle of the month, we went skiing with friends in southern Sweden for a few days. The kids had never tried it before and quickly fell in love with it. It was bittersweet for me – after a skateboarding injury sustained while trying to keep up with them a few years ago, I was not risking life and limb again. But I craved the colours white and deep green, so I came along for the ride.

I waved the family off at the door of our rented cabin and started to plot my own route. While they were hurtling down the snowy slopes, I was going bathing, only this time it was not in the sea. I was heading to the forest.

This type of bathing is one that you do with your clothes on: it's all about immersion in the woods, rather than immersion in water. It's quite simple. To begin with, you walk slowly along the forest track under the trees and tune into your five senses. Think about what you can see, what you can smell, what you can touch, what you can hear and what the air tastes like when you breathe in. Breathe deeply a few times and look around closely with curiosity. Be completely in the moment. And leave your mobile phone and camera behind. Don't let the simplicity of this approach fool you: it has a proven impact on mental health.

Shinrin-yoku, or forest bathing, was developed in 1980s Japan as an antidote to the tech-boom burnout. I am old enough to remember how space age and futuristic Japan felt when I was growing up, the land of Donkey Kong and kawaii and tech innovations like that yellow Sony Walkman I craved when I was ten. The fact that doctor and researcher Qing Li discovered that just being in nature could reduce your stress levels and blood pressure 40 years ago, and that Japanese tech workers needed it, showed just how far ahead they were.

The full set of benefits included not just those physiological markers, but mental health benefits too: forest bathing can improve your feelings of happiness, boost your immune system, speed up your recovery from illness or infection, increase vigour, reduce fatigue, help you sleep and boost your creativity. In that, it shares some similarities with cold-water swimming. It's all the things I wanted and needed right then; I thought about how sad it is that our tech-guided daily lives are more convenient, but at the same time lead us away from the things we need most, the rhythms, colours and sounds of nature. Too much of one and not enough of the other can lead to a sense of burnout where you can only recover through intensive sessions in nature.

I read about what you had to do in the forest to get these benefits, and it seemed it was more about what you didn't do that mattered. While you can book sessions with forest-bathing practitioners to lead you in mindfulness meditations and guided walks, you don't have to. This, like swimming, is something you can do on your own, with friends, whenever you want. There's no specialist kit to buy and no one to tell you you're falling behind or not doing it right. I'll be honest, I would have gone swimming if I had been able to, but the nearest lake was half covered with ice and had a muddy beach that looked forbidding. And that word 'bathing' sounded hugely appealing. I wanted to be wrapped up in nature, dunked in it up to my shoulders, to sink my feet into the mud and be part of something bigger than myself, something that didn't care what I earned or what my future plans were, that was here, right now, and living.

As much as 69 per cent of Sweden is covered in forest, and the vast majority of that is coniferous, with pine in the north and spruce and birch in the south. Half of Sweden's forests are privately owned, but thanks to the Right of Public Access, or *allemans-rätten*, everyone has the right to roam the countryside in Sweden. You can walk, cycle, ski and camp on any land except in private gardens, or near a dwelling, a house or on land under cultivation. It also means that you can collect flowers, mushrooms and berries, drive on private roads (unless a sign says otherwise), swim in lakes and access any beach as long as you stay away from private residences. As I pulled on my hat and gloves, it was a relief to know that there would be no farmer waving his 10-bore at me and bellowing at me to 'get off his land'.

This right to roam comes with a few responsibilities: you have to take care of nature and wildlife, and show consideration for landowners and other people enjoying the countryside. Put succinctly, the Swedish Environmental Protection Agency (EPA) just says, 'Don't disturb – don't destroy'.

While forest bathing is a Japanese practice, it has been making its way around the world. Scandinavia is a prime place to practise it. It's also a culture with a deep love of fresh air and outdoor living, its hallowed *friluftsliv*. When I mentioned forest bathing to a Danish friend, she looked at me strangely as if to say, Why put labels and research on something we all know to be true? Fresh air, nature and work–life balance are the key ingredients to a good life here anyway.

I wanted to find out more about forest bathing and how people practised it in Scandinavia, so I called Thuri Kledal, a Nordic forest-bathing guide and the founder and CEO of NaturRefugium, one of Denmark's primary forest-bathing centres. She spent years training to be a forest therapist, including time spent studying in Japan, and has developed a strand of Nordic nature therapy in Denmark over the last thirteen years.

'The thing to realise,' she said, 'is that we don't have the same nature or culture as they do in Japan so you have to take a different approach. It's critical to take the practice and include your own culture so you can grasp and own it. I take a more animistic [the belief that natural objects, natural phenomena and the universe itself possess souls] way of looking at it, a more Nordic way of looking at nature as giving us signs, which goes back to the Norse gods. It adds a different dimension.'

Before you think it, Thuri isn't into crystals and healing stones. Far from it – she had a professional background working with medical devices, an MSc and a PhD, and is a certified eco-therapist, working with the evidence-based effects of nature on relaxation. She leads nature therapy and forest bathing sessions and also trains new therapists. She guides walks and leads therapy sessions in Denmark's forests, meadows and seashores, and says that it's an interesting place to do it.

'In the last few years, we've seen a rise and then a fall in interest in forest bathing. There's still a huge gap between what people think it is and what it is. They think it's a walk in a forest – some people think it's swimming in a lake in a forest – but it's much more than that. It's very important to activate the senses, both the primary and the secondary ones.

'I'm always humble about what happens when I go into nature with my clients,' she continues. 'We start by grounding ourselves, then use our senses and introduce ourselves to different issues. I don't always know the depth of their problem and they may not either. I'm there to facilitate and guide how nature affects them – and we find the most remarkable insights. We walk through and ask nature for an answer to their hardest questions. It might seem strange but most clients are amazed about what they get back. Often they see a sign, perhaps there's something in their way as they are walking, and we stop and look at it to see if it tells them something. Most of the time they discover the root of the problem and are really moved.

'For me, it's a goosebump-making moment when that happens. It can become close to spiritual for many people. It's this thread back to the animistic way of looking at nature, looking for signs. It's your own subconscious making it conscious.'

Forget Thuri's goosebumps, I've got goosebumps of my own just thinking about it. It goes deeper than belief, however – and it's important to Thuri and to me that this isn't just a branch of spiritual woo-woo, but has a basis in science and research. Forest bathing and its impact has been the subject of scientific research in Japan and is in active use as a therapeutical practice in the UK and Australia as well. However, to date, Nordic forest bathing is still a little light on specific research about the physiological benefits relating to the tree varieties available here.

'We're also still waiting for research about phytoncides in mid-European forests to be completed – we aren't able to prove that forest bathing can help against cancer or even how seasonal changes affect the phytoncides you're exposed to in our forests,' she said. 'The cedar tree in Japan is singular as part of the forest bathing experience, but we don't have them here. It is critical to choose places where you have the right trees. How do birch and oak work together? Oak trees, especially in autumn, have a scent. Does it have a chemical effect? We don't know yet.'

I was intrigued by the practice and by Thuri herself. As we chatted, it turned out that we had a few things in common. Her path to running this unique establishment started thirteen years ago, when she broke free from a successful job and corporate life in search of something that would suit her better. A single mum, she longed to give her son the life she had as a child, when she spent afternoons roaming in her nearby forest with her father. She rearranged her job so she could have a more flexible schedule, allowing her to embrace forest walks in the afternoon, and eventually broke free altogether so she could expand on the sensory experiences she'd had as a child and create a restorative process from it.

In her final job, the stimuli from the huge open-plan office, all the phone noise, conversations and screens, became too much. I could certainly relate. She knew she wanted to do something else and took her biggest passion of being in nature and found a way to help others and to help herself at the same time, starting on a journey where she could train and gain certification and move into something that made sense to the deeper parts of herself. It was a journey I couldn't help but admire. I wondered a little about whether I was doing the right thing – maybe I should be taking my passion about swimming and making that into something too? But I didn't want to be a swimming teacher, and I wasn't sure being a lifeguard was for me either. I thought about whether I also needed a big change, like her.

Her thoughts about the nerve-jangling nature of an open-plan office really resonated with me. I never felt like I could quite be myself in the office, and I never felt like my time was really mine. Even if I had a schedule and ten or so sticky notes on my desk marking out my priorities for the day and week ahead, there was always someone ready to pull me aside, drop by my desk or tell me that their project was more important. If I was going to have a career change, it would have to be one where I could have control of my time and the pace at which I worked. Trying to work with my natural rhythms, like the sea, like the forest, seemed to make absolute sense in my head, even if it wouldn't make sense to a project manager. I know I'm more focused in the morning, and better at admin in the afternoon. I knew my best ideas came before 11am. So maybe there was a way to harness that knowledge and turn back to something that felt natural to me. It was something to keep thinking about.

We had another thing in common, too – both of our names are connected to trees. Just like a Norwegian mountain guide I met in Bergen back in November called Turid, Thuri's name derives from the Old Norse for Thor, the god of thunder. He was not just the god of thunder, though – he was also the god of oak trees. As for me, Laura is derived from 'laurel'. Not such a mighty tree, in some eyes more of a shrub, but I was going to call it a tree anyway.

I started my walk down the long track into the pine forest from the isolated country cottage we were staying in, with just my dog Max for company. We passed two small copses on the left, edged by leafless silver birch trees looking brittle and skeletal before the impossibly tall spruce trees, crowns waving in the breeze. Once we were in the forest, all I could see was green.

There is a peculiar quality to a Swedish forest, something I'd noticed before, that makes it feel like you could stumble on fairies, or a council of wolves, or a portal to another dimension. There's a feeling of something ancient, something trapped in time, to it. It's the height of the trees, for a start, which would tower over an English forest the way that New York skyscrapers would dominate a typical market town. It's also the moss that covers every surface, like a wall-to-wall green shagpile carpet from the 1970s. It's deep and soft and your feet sink into it without a sound.

In a deciduous forest you might find mud on the ground and leaves all over it in differing states of decay, but in a pine forest, the leaves mostly stay on the trees, with just shattered twigs of pine needles blown off in the wind making it to the ground. The moss covers everything: boulders, tree roots, tree stumps and the banks of streams. It acts like soundproofing in a recording studio, damping down the sounds, while the tall trees block out light.

Strain your ears for sound and you'll hear a roaring, rushing noise from the treetops as their crowns brush against each other in the breeze; an occasional creak from an inflexible trunk, and perhaps a pee-whit of a bird. Most of the birds are higher in the canopy so you can't see or hear them. To an English ear, the forest seems unnervingly quiet.

At ground level, there is a slow fight for survival for every seed that falls from the smooth armadillo-scaled pinecones onto the moss. With towering grandfathers and great grandfathers above them, Christmas tree-sized spruces are fighting for light. If they've got this far, they've already seen off the challenges of deer nibbling their tender shoots and now stand waiting for a gale to fell an old soldier and give them a pure patch of light to grow up and into.

If they don't make it, the moss will claim them and the tree will mulch the forest floor to provide energy for the fungal systems that connect the forest underground, as well as insects and more. It all creates a multidisciplinary life cycle where everything is critical to everything else – a community of a sort – and at the end of it all, everything is weighed down with moss.

The path was wet with pockets of snow here and there, but in drier patches, pinecones were sprung like the hackles of a threatened cat. A frond of the palest green lichen, fruticose lichen I thought, common in arctic forests, clung to a fallen pine shoot.

I touched it, expecting brittleness, but found a gummy resilience. It reminded me of the texture of dried-up UPVC glue, a pliable soft plastic, and I was taken back to when I was eight and we bought packs of lichen just like these from a model railway shop to use as lifelike bushes around the edge of a castle in topic week at school. I brought myself back to the moment.

Rain started falling – suddenly this was a different sort of forest bathing – and I sheltered under a tree until the worst passed. I watched droplets of rain caught on the needles of a pine frond, bulging at the end before they dripped. Max sat, expectantly. Next to us, rain fell, creating neat concentric circles into the standing water of a ditch. In a few months, the ditches here would be wriggling with tadpoles, and months further on, pulsing with midge larvae. Time in Sweden has taught me that insect repellent is a necessity – and that you should always, always check for ticks.

The rain faltered and we walked on. We passed stony tracks leading to nowhere. Trees thinned and I could see through them to a meadow with a little red cabin, the size of a caravan, perched in the middle. *Sommarstuga* are these simple little red-painted huts you find all over Scandinavia, called *sommarhus* in Danish and *sommerhytte* in Norwegian. They are sometimes called 'holiday cottages', but that term always puts me in mind of an achingly pretty but overpriced stone cottage somewhere in Cornwall with a view of the sea, so the translation never quite fits for me. Here in northern Europe, these holiday cottages are used for holidays, so that part is right, but they tend to have more basic facilities, rather than cupboards of Cornishware and a restored Aga to enjoy. Walls tend to be thin and almost shed-like, and it may be more accurate to say that they are a beach hut, inexplicably placed in the middle of a field, perhaps with a view of a lake, but certainly a long way from a high-tide mark.

They are a well-worn tradition, largely because they offer that distinct escape into nature. In Finland, one in five people own a summerhouse, and the rest of the population rent them, so they can take their own trips to the countryside to bathe in lakes and forests and restore their natural balance. This little cottage looked idyllic, perched in a meadow that would be full of flowers in a few months, and surrounded on two sides by forest.

I picked up a pine frond and sniffed it tentatively. It didn't smell of anything. I half wondered if I had a problem with my sense of smell before I remembered the scent comes from the sap in the trunk, not the needles. I cast it aside.

The more I walk, the more I'm reminded of how different the woods of Scandinavia are to the English woods where I grew up. They seem grander and more austere, less human in so many ways, and so much taller. Woodlands in England seem to have a children's picture-book quality to them, where you can imagine the Magic Faraway Tree growing, just one super-tall tree in the forest rather than many.

They've always had a bit of a spell over me. Once in a forest south of Bristol, my husband and I took our unruly toddler for a Sunday walk in ancient woodlands and saw, for a golden moment, a fallow deer spotlit by a shaft of sunlight in a clearing. It stood still, looked at us with big liquid eyes, then hopped over a log and went on its way. It was like a scene from a medieval painting, or a momentary slip through time to the 1500s, and something peculiarly English. When I think of magical woods, I think of moments like those.

I don't feel any of that here. While there are deer, elk and foxes in the southern Swedish forests and Max had already caused a large hare to go leaping off across moss-covered boulders, its black and white tail flashing, there is nothing of the human perspective in a vast pine forest. Trees are too high to climb. Hundred-year-old stone cottages are reduced to mossy lumps. Footprints erase. The human gaze is nothing when things are happening on a far grander scale altogether.

I watched the tips of the pine trees sway, moving metres with the wind while their thin trunks flexed. According to reports and studies by the likes of the World Health Organization,* people feel the most relaxed when looking at the colours of blue and green. There were so many colours of green here – the

* World Health Organization, 'Green and Blue Spaces and Mental Health: New Evidence and Perspectives for Action', 2021: https://iris.who.int/bitstream/handle/10665/342931/9789289055666-eng.pdf

minty green of grass, a brilliant yellow-green moss, a deeper green star-shaped brush plant, the palest white-green bearded lichen growing from branches. Pine needles went from mid to dark green as the shadows fell. All was green.

The researcher who initiated the forest medicine movement, Qing Li, discovered forest bathing while he was a stressed-out medical student. It reminded me that I used to pack a bag of papers and books and head to the lido in Oxford to revise and relax in my final year at university, because the swimming calmed me down and laps helped me cement those facts and theories better than anything else. Just bathing, never mind the forest, has always been helpful.

Max was looking bedraggled and kept stopping, so as more rain started to fall, we turned and headed back to the cottage. I was surprised and a little disappointed that I hadn't seen any deer or elk in the forest. I only found a strange round snow-coloured stone that fitted beautifully in the palm of my hand. I stashed it in my pocket and promised myself I'd return at dusk when the elk might be more active. The thought of encountering a long-limbed elk in the forest was at once exciting and terrifying, just as a connection with the ancients and the natural lore of the land should be. I might be a city lover but I can't resist the pull of these kinds of stories. I wanted to wrap myself in its green legends, even here, where the trees threatened to dwarf and overwhelm me at every turn.

I stopped on the edge of the forest to take five deep lungfuls of forest air. It was clear and cold and clean. Then we walked back to the cottage as the sun broke the grey-white sky into clouds.

There was no doubt in my mind that setting a course for swimming my way out of burnout was doing me good and helping me move forward, and bathing in the woods, in lieu of anywhere to swim, was working too, while I took the time to set up my great Scandinavian swimming adventure plan. But after this break in Sweden, I could see that the stillness of the forest added something richer to my Scandinavian experience. I determined to add forest bathing to my recovery plan as well.

Later, as the sun started to sink behind the trees, I walked slowly along the edge of the field at the back of the cottage looking for hoofprints. I only found my own clumsy snow boot prints. But then, in a nest in the slippery snowmelt-rich grass, I found handfuls of oval-shaped elk droppings. I hadn't been alone in the forest after all.

10

When I started thinking about constructing a swimming journey around Scandinavia and the Nordics, there was one country that I knew had to be part of the plan: Iceland. This volcanic, windswept island in the North Atlantic has swimming at its core, thanks to its natural hot springs. In Iceland, you can't graduate school until you have learned to swim. In Iceland, the equivalent of the pub is the hot tub, a place to mix with locals and chat about life. A swimming mission in Scandinavia and Northern Europe had to include Iceland as a bare minimum. And I needed a special local guide. I found Kristín Jórunn Hjartardóttir on Instagram, a fellow winter bather but with a far more exotic edge. In the land of the geothermal hot springs, she swims just about everywhere else, in the freezing North Atlantic Ocean.

Kristín is an icon for me in many ways, and not just because she is lovely. When she turned 60, she decided to swim in 60 cold water spots around Iceland to celebrate, calling the project '60iscool' and to document it on her feed. She's since turned it into a book, with pictures by her photographer husband, that charts these extraordinary swimming spots on the furthest edges of Europe. As a travel journalist who has written a lot about Reykjavik and Iceland in the past, I knew a lot about the local geothermal pools. The sea around the island, though, not so much.

I called her to find out where the idea came from, and what it's been like to swim around the outside of the country, not just the inside. Sat radiating goodness and energy in her Reykjavik home, with long silver hair, Kristín looked just like a mermaid on my computer screen.

She first tried cold-water swimming in the North Atlantic seven years ago, and was not an immediate convert.

'It was horrible!' she said. 'I was always a super active person and was always running, so I thought I'd try swimming. But while it wasn't what I was expecting – really, it was horrible – there was still a feeling inside me that made me think: yeah, I'll do that again. I haven't stopped swimming since.'

The swimming-around-Iceland project started as Kristín approached a milestone birthday. But while many of us might think about throwing a party, she was thinking bigger.

'When I turned 59, I thought, *Oh, I'm going to be 60 next year – I have to do something about it!*' she said. 'So along with my photographer partner, now husband, I have been swimming in lovely places around Iceland. Sixty is not so old these days, anyway.'

As well as swimming three times a week in Reykjavik, she has now swum in over 90 locations around the country. Kristín's local spot is Nautholsvik Beach, the man-made beach in the city of Reykjavik itself.

As we swapped tales of swimming and sea life, and talked about how we prefer not to swim in a wetsuit, I couldn't help but feel great admiration for her and her pursuits. Even in her favourite swimming spot, the iceberg-crowded Jokulsarlon, a lagoon at the foot of a glacier in South Iceland, Kristín just wore a swimsuit, gloves and swim socks – no wetsuit to be seen. For her, it's all about the endorphins she gets afterwards. After swimming in so many cold places, the feeling is still not undimmed for her, something that puts me at ease. I was wondering if your body gets used to it and if that natural high, that addictive rush, eases with time, but she said it was alive and kicking for her.

It's not just a case of chasing the feeling of having been in the water that fuels her – it's also about feeling a connection with nature.

'You can't get much closer connection with nature than swimming in the sea in clean cold water,' she said. 'You can walk on land, but in the water you are surrounded and connected with nature. I can't describe the feeling in English but it's the one true thing for me.'

I felt it too. Somehow swimming in the cold saltwater is about something deeper than just activity or keeping fit. It was not just about swimming, otherwise we'd all get this feeling from a local swimming pool. It was not just about challenging ourselves, otherwise we'd get it from the gym. There was just this little magic component that nature brings which makes it different.

I remembered back to the trip I took to Bergen, where I met Linn and started my pledge to swim every week in the harbour. That day, we also hiked a mountain just outside the city, with a Norwegian nature guide called Turid. We had been talking about how the mountains in Bergen were used in years gone by, and how women had not been able to access them for a long time because their big skirts and footwear made them too difficult to climb. We talked about whether men and women experienced nature differently today, and she said she thought they did. According to her, women liked to be in nature, and men liked to compete in nature.

I thought it was really interesting, and perhaps it shed some light on to why there seemed to be so many women winter swimming versus men (though, of course, men and women can both do it, there are no rules). Perhaps the lack of competition – apart from maybe with yourself about how long you can stay in for – is something that makes a difference. It's more about being part of nature and being connected than jostling for any kind of podium.

I wondered how different the experience of swimming in Iceland was from swimming further south in the Nordics. I asked Kristín if she had seen more fish in the water, or perhaps seals or whales? Kristín laughed, and told me about the time a curious seal swam up to her and it really scared her. We talked about the great lion's mane jellyfish, and how we really didn't want to be stung by them, about the fish we see in the water, and then she told me about one time when she went swimming in a bay with a strange whale-smell to it. It wasn't until she came out that she saw the rotting carcass of a whale, exposed ribs, blackening blubber and all, a little way along on the sand, where it had been towed by the local council to decay naturally away from the more popular places.

A couple of strong ideas stood out to me as she talked about how swimming had changed her. It had changed how she looked at the landscape of Iceland – when she was travelling around her country, she found that it was no longer a landscape of volcanoes and glaciers, but a patchwork of hot pools and thermal rivers, lakes, harbours and beaches. Her eyes were always seeking the pathways down to the sea and the easiest way to slip into the water and become part of it. She also said that way back when she started all of this, she was in a toxic relationship and was depressed. Swimming gave her a burst, unlocked something inside of her and made her happy. She said it was the best thing she'd done in her life.

I didn't doubt it for one minute. As we said our goodbyes to each other, I felt that fizz of electricity I got from swimming rising in my blood, just from talking to her about it. Good things happen when swimming ladies get together. *If I am lucky enough to make it to Iceland this year,* I thought, *I know who I'll call first.*

11

As spring hovered on the horizon, I was in a buoyant mood. I was swimming two or three times a week in the coldest water I'd ever been in, with two regular swimming buddies, and I was even looking forward to it. In the morning, I slipped into my swimming costume and wore it under my clothes as I walked the kids and the dog to school, then rushed back to leave the dog at home and grabbed a couple of towels as I headed down to the water to jump in.

I was fizzing with energy. Happiness bubbled up out of nowhere. Hanna noted that I'd taken over from her as the keenest swimmer of the three of us. It was natural that we would take turns – that's why we'd banded together, after all – because we wouldn't always feel like we wanted to and the pull of the group kept us going. But I had noticed the extreme cold was having a positive effect – even on -1°C mornings, I didn't hesitate to climb down the ladder and into the water. I wasn't afraid of what would happen or whether I could cope with it. I walked home from the harbour like I was walking on air, my skin charged, feeling truly alive. I couldn't wait to swim again.

It was only my seventh week of properly committing to swimming once a week, and my fourth month of winter swimming overall. The winter would last here for at least another two months, teasing us with sunny days and then drenching us and blasting us with freezing winds until it relaxed into a new mode in May. It had taken me a while to get into the rhythms of the Danish seasons, and now in my fifth year, I was starting to see a regularity to it, a pace that differed from life in England. There is a noticeable lack of spring and autumn, for a start. Spring blends into winter rather than being a quarter of the year as I've thought of it in England. Daffodils bloom on traffic islands for a couple of weeks and the pharmacy windows are plastered with adverts for treatments for hay fever caused by the birch pollen. Then you wake up one day and it's summer.

I was excited about the coming spring. It might not have been coming as quickly as I'd have liked, but I knew it was on the way when I found a lone snowdrop plant growing in a terracotta pot in the courtyard. It was under a month to the spring equinox – and positive change was on the way.

Change was coming in me as well. A spurt of atypical confidence welled up out of nowhere and I spoke to my friends in confident Danish. To their credit, they didn't laugh or even raise their eyebrows. Something was finally going right.

Remarkable as it seemed to me, work was starting to come together too. I began to plan ways that I could use my skills outside of a classic office environment and still make it work. I helped small businesses with projects and had coffee meetings all over town to try to build a network and gather stories that I could pitch to newspapers and websites. The confidence boost was carrying through to that part of my life too, the part where I would show up in a café, introduce myself and feel that far from being a washed-up quitter who couldn't hold on to a corporate job, I was someone with something to offer.

Since embarking on this journey, I'd been extra conscious about how limited time was. Perhaps it's a post-COVID realisation, or a note on what it is to be growing older, with children who throw your age into relief every day that passes. It seemed to me that none of us have unlimited time to do the things we want to do, and that the most in-demand commodity I had was time, not money. I started to think about doing more meaningful work, and found it made sense. Instead of being passive, I'd be active: I'd speak up and say what I thought might be a better and more effective plan, or just plain suggest something I thought would be great to do. It worked: I started to do more and more of what I wanted to do, to write more and more stories about the things that made my heart pound. I put it down to what was happening in the water: I now had more experience of actively chasing things that made me feel good and I was starting to get used to it. The cold-water swimming spilled over into other areas, making me braver, more able to say no, and more attuned to what I wanted to do and what made me happy. I felt like I'd taken some power back, and I started to think: *If I can do that, what else can I do?*

I swam twice in two days, once alone apart from a pair of ducks slowly tracing the waves under the bridge, and once with Hanna and Sonia, where I stayed in for longer than ever before. The water was a bracing 4.2°C and the air was even colder. My skin was burning afterwards and I was all lit up inside for the rest of the day. A storm passed by the day before and another was on the horizon. The water level in the canals and city harbour rose.

While I was still swimming regularly in Copenhagen, the ideas about swimming in Scandinavia were growing. I'd pinpointed places I wanted to visit, adding to my Pinterest board new natural spring spas in Iceland, seawater pools with saunas in Finland and the clean harbour of Oslo, with its rows of sauna boats lined up to help you warm up after a dip. Now that I was looking, all kinds of ideas were emerging about where I could swim and who with. I wasn't quite sure how I was going to pull it off, but I thought that maybe the more work I did as a writer in Scandinavia, the more it would happen naturally. If I was sent to Stockholm to write about something, all I'd have to do was put a swimsuit in my bag and give myself an extra few hours in the city to find somewhere to swim. It wasn't that hard, now that everything was set up.

In the afternoon after my swim with Hanna and Sonia, great blobs of wet snow fell to remind me that we were still in February and winter was not going out quietly. Still, I felt hope. Somehow, the dark heart of winter seemed to have been pierced. The mornings were just slightly lighter and the evenings a fraction longer. You could smell the change of the season in the air. I started to think about swimming in the summer, and about how I'd swim every morning and every evening. I might even swim across the harbour from Teglholmen, the island I live on, to Sluseholmen, the next island over, connected by a bridge and only a few hundred metres away. I'd swim laps in the pool at Fisketorvet and in the bigger pool at Islands Brygge. I'd dive into the sea at Kastrup Sea Bath. My hair would dry in the sun in the time it took to walk from the floating swimming pool a few streets away back home to my sun-filled flat.

The change of seasons brought on a new challenge: cluster headaches. I'd been suffering from these since my mid-twenties, a chain of headaches best described as a stabbing pain like a cramp in one side of the head. It causes your nose to run, your eye to throb and the whole side of your face, including your gums, to pulse in pain. Being in a space with any light at all is intensely painful. They have the intensity of a migraine headache, except they are only on one side of the face, for me always the same side, and they only last about 20 minutes. The kicker is that it lasts for 20 minutes every day, often the same time each day, for up to 30 days in a row. It's enough to drive you mad.

I hadn't had cluster headaches for years – they can disappear and reappear again – but my heart sank as soon as I started to feel that familiar throb behind my right eye. *Here we go again.*

I normally used a SAD light during the winter because I'd regularly found the super-dark mornings affected my mood, but I'd been so busy I hadn't used it for a couple of weeks. Probably, it seems to me, that had upset the balance and my brain was now acting out. I spent a weekend in and out of dark rooms and resigned myself to it for another few weeks. My body was forcing me to slow down and pace myself – that wasn't such a bad thing.

Being rusty in how to treat it, I looked it up and saw that these headaches are frequently brought on by the changing length of days and can be a seasonal thing. For years I had thought they were brought on by stress, chocolate or coffee, but as I raked back through my memory, they were always a feature of early spring or early autumn, and it suddenly made sense. My own private equinox detector. I was more in tune with the seasons that I realised. How very Scandinavian of me. It's always seemed to me that Scandinavians have a finer sensor about the dark and the light to us Brits, and that they undergo a behaviour shift from spring to summer, becoming more gregarious, and from autumn to winter with a kind of hibernation. They mark Midsummer in a much more impressive way, with crayfish parties and bonfires, and the winter equinox as well. There is a very different gear change when the season changes, and people cast off their grey, brown and black winter clothes to wear colour and floral prints in the summer. Days are longer and the pace changes accordingly, with evening strolls and picnics on bridges. It's a visual shift and it's everywhere. It's another way to be in touch with nature and the outside world, instead of trying to live every day as if it's exactly the same, like a robot. I was all for it, but it was a real pain all the same.

One gloomy Thursday evening, I met Hanna at a pop-up floating sauna in the city for a *saunagus*. I'd never known what this word meant – I'd seen it on adverts and flyers at the swimming pool, and wasn't sure how it was different from a sauna. I was about to find out.

The pop-up floating sauna was a novelty too: a box-like modern sauna made from wood with big picture windows, sat atop a floating wooden raft and tethered to one side of the canal next to the Stromma boat-tour stop. Inside, there was a small changing area with lockable cubbies, a door to the sauna, with space for up to eight people, and a digital thermostat on the wall that said 58°C. A friend had told me that sometimes it got as hot as 80°C in a *saunagus*, and I didn't know if she was joking with me or not. By the look of it, probably not. I shoved my rucksack into a locker and stripped off quickly, prepared for the heat.

The *saunagus* is a sauna ritual run by a sauna master, who, over the course of the session, pours aromatherapy oils on the sauna, wafts them around in the air with a towel or special fan, with mood lighting and gentle music in the background. It takes place several times – for us, three times in an hour – with a break after fifteen minutes to exit the sauna, stand on the deck in the cold Copenhagen night air, be photographed by passing tourists on the low-lying Stromma canal boat tour, and, if you're feeling daring, to tip a bucket of extremely cold water all over you.

Sweat ran down my neck and cleavage and on to the benches. I was a jockey, sweating down to the right weight, a middleweight boxer trying to lose enough kilos to perform as a welterweight. Rivulets of sweat coursed down my pink thighs. Outside, the canal's eddies shone in the moonlight while high in the sky, two neon green search lights made a cross in the sky above Christiansborg Palace, the seat of the Danish Parliament, as part of the city's Festival of Light. God knows we needed light in February – at 6pm, it was pitch black. Red brake lights shone on the wet cobbles, and up in the palace building, lights started going out until there were just a handful on the third and fourth floors. The sauna master shushed us, encouraging us instead to focus on the cedarwood, vetiver and blood orange scents.

Saunagus rules state that it's not a place to chat. It's a serious business, all this sweating.

I thought about the longing I had to go swimming in Finland before the spring came. I had hoped to make a pilgrimage to the home of winter bathing, right back to the source, where people build a sauna before they build their house, and generations had been born into saunas and enjoyed the cycle of cold-water swimming and steamy heating sessions before me. Spring comes late in Helsinki, and I had thought an early break in the Finnish capital could give me a chance to see how truly brave I really was, with an ice bath. There's a floating swimming pool in Helsinki harbour too, where the water is heated, and that was always an option if the icy lake was too much.

At the first break, we stumbled outside and I poured the wooden bucket of cold water all over me. It took my breath away, but as soon as we were back inside, I warmed up in an instant. Looking to the side of the floating raft, green lights shone underwater. It was too rough to see them clearly, but there were mermaids and mermen in this part of the harbour. A mermaid and seven mermen, to be exact – it's a sculpture celebrating the legend of Agnete and the Merman, a folk tale about a woman who went to live with a merman. She bore him seven sons, and lived happily under the water until one day she heard church bells ringing and felt a calling to go back to her family. When she made it back to them, she discovered that the church bells were ringing for the death of her father. She stayed on land, forsaking her sons and mer-husband, much to their great sadness, and the sculpture shows her breaking away from them as they beg her to stay.

There's a bittersweetness to the tale – the heartbreak of being from another world really resonates when you're a foreigner and have a foot in two countries. I miss, sometimes, talking to people who have known me for more than a few years, and a lifetime of shared TV shows and cultural references. I don't often get homesick, but I think I will always miss Marks & Spencer, Marmite and Twinings tea. But you'd be surprised, too, how many Danes know *Fawlty Towers* off by heart, or can discuss the finer points of an episode of *Midsomer Murders*.

It had been a good week – an ordinary one, by most standards – and I felt positive about what was around the corner, despite the looming war. Crocuses were pushing up their yellow trumpets in the grass beside the main roads, and in the morning I walked the dog mindfully, taking in crispy brown oak leaves on the nearby trees, round buds bulging on others, and two bluetits perched on top of a tall bare tree, tweeting to each other before flying off into the wind. I'd been lucky enough to meet a bunch of new people in a work-related event one evening and start a program with them as a mentor for the first time, and I felt quite excited about it all. I knew that three things make me really happy – being creative, swimming and meeting new people – and I'd been able to do all of them this week.

I'm not saying I was recovered. I was not sure I was even halfway to finding the better life that I was seeking. But I did know that it was possible to intentionally curate and create a life that made more sense and bred more happiness. Following those three things that I knew worked seemed like an easy rule of thumb.

Where the start of February had felt like falling down a long dark hole, as I reached the end of March, I could see some light. I celebrated with a second swim at the Snegl in Kastrup on a bright sunny afternoon. Above me, a chiselled man in pink Bermudas swallow dived off the high board, while I swam breaststroke off the seaweedy steps, sending ripples into the water ahead and behind me. After him, another naked man hurled himself into the water. I wondered if it was the same naked man as last time, or if every time I swam here, there would be an exhibitionist male in the buff at the ready.

12

I'd been seeing a Frenchman who lived in Nørrebro, the hippest quarter of Copenhagen, a lot lately. Gaël was pretty unique, and I'd found that the more I swam, the more I met people with an interesting story to tell. His started during the COVID lockdown, when a friend dared him to build a floating sauna in Copenhagen harbour.

He downloaded open-source plans from Canada showing how to build one, and when lumber arrived in the autumn, things got serious. What had felt like a fun plan, a flight of fancy for the underemployed engineer and his friend, became reality in the rain of November and the dark afternoons of December. It became clear it wasn't a project that would be completed in a week or two: the dark, cold and windy winter months were full of sawing and hammering without a workshop or a shelter. A lesser person would have given up. But not him.

He built a raft, then a cabin. Added a wood-burning sauna. Checked it floated and checked again. Wrangled with the local harbour authorities about where to moor it. Then finally launched it. All winter it had been moored in the harbour just a few streets from where I lived. He was usually the one there greeting people as they dropped by for an hour-long sauna and dip session, standing in an irrepressibly French way, making everything look a little bit chicer.

As saunas go, it wasn't perfect. Depending on how many people were crammed into its small box-like sauna cabin, and whether the weight distribution was right or not, it might list a little to the side. The door, which had expanded a little thanks to the exposure to steam and sweat, sometimes jammed in an alarming way. But I liked the spirit of it, the idea that you could decide to do something a little off plan and make it work anyway. Kasia, Hanna and I booked sessions, late in the evening during the week or on a lazy Sunday, a chance to escape the dark nights and do something other than watch TV, and a definite aid to swimming in these parts in the winter. Regular saunas are good for you, for your blood pressure and for your mental health, acting like tiny community rooms where people of all walks of life can come together. The experience had me thinking of Finland, home of the sauna, and the great floating swimming pool in Helsinki harbour that I'd seen and wanted so very much to visit. On dark winter mornings I imagined early morning swimmers taking laps in the semi-heated open-air pool in the harbour, their breath and the warmth spiralling into the icy air. Helsinki was only around a two-hour flight away: it seemed possible, likely even, that I would go swimming there one day, and maybe one day soon.

By chance, I was put in touch with Ylva Watkins, a Finnish swimmer based in the Åland islands, and we chatted one dark late winter night about a delightful informal swimming group she and her friends had created: The Åland Lighthouse Swimmers. It was what it sounds like – a group of women who swim around the lighthouses of the Åland islands off the southwest tip of Finland.

It started innocently enough, as these things do – the group of women aged 40–55 were swimming regularly in local swimming pools and decided to train for a bigger challenge: open-water swimming.

'One of the group knew someone with a boat, and there are a lot of lighthouses here in the Åland islands, so it seemed the natural next step,' she explained. 'We've done the best-known ones around here and so far have swum around three or four lighthouses.'

It sounded like a charming challenge, but when you think a little more about it and what a lighthouse is for, and where it is located, it was far from easy. Positioned to warn ships about not coming too close to land, in places where there can be dangerous rocks and waves, it's a long way from swimming laps of the local pool.

'It can be really dangerous,' she admitted, 'and when you're out in the sea it can be a bit scary at times. The waves can be so high that you can't always see the other swimmers so you're quite alone. The water changes a lot as well, so you have very calm inlets and sometimes it's so shallow you have to stand.'

The group swims in wetsuits with fins and a floatation device so they can be seen, and have made this a summer pursuit, since being in the water for such a long time in the cold waters at other times of year up in Finland is often not possible. This pursuit, like most open-water swimming, is weather-dependent too, and relies on the friend with the boat and accurate weather forecasts the night before, as well as finding time away from work and family.

The team aspect of the challenge is important as well – you're never alone, as she says, and you have to take responsibility for yourself and the others. It's not a race – and Ylva would know, having swum in open-water races herself. For her, it's not about winning anything, it's about doing something different, creating a new challenge and a new path that can be forged with a group of friends, together.

'The first time was really amazing,' she said. 'The water changed as we rounded the lighthouse, with high waves on one side and calm on the other. The adrenaline rush you get from it is incredible. I felt really high at the end.'

There are plenty more lighthouses for the swimmers to add to their list, but right now it's winter and they are all training indoors until the summer swings by. I think about whether I'd ever feel strong enough to swim round a lighthouse in rough seas, when you can't see over the tops of the waves and are lost amid a sea of water, until you see a friend's bright float and your feelings of fear and fight are overcome as you swim back, around the calmer side of the rocks, together. It feels scary but vital at the same time.

Talking to all these amazing swimming women started a chain of thoughts: about going to the Arctic Circle to swim, and about what it might be like to dip a toe in the water in Greenland. Could I swim the Hellespont, like Lord Byron, or the Øresund Strait from Denmark to Sweden? I haven't ever swum competitively in open water, but then again, I hadn't swum in the sea in winter like this before. Great possibilities were opening up.

I calculated how many laps of the local swimming pool I would have to be able to swim to cover the shortest distance from Denmark to Sweden, eight kilometres. Since each lap of the uniquely round public swimming pool was approximately 100 metres, it would only be 80 circuits of the pool. 'Only'. For reference, I usually swam 10–15 rounds when I visited. The Hellespont was less, 4.5 kilometres, with an assist from the current that reputedly makes it easier. I wondered what other currents I could feel, and what other seas I could experience. How would they feel on my skin? Who was swimming in them, and why?

III. Spring

13

After some months of swimming in Denmark, it was high time I started the Scandinavian swim adventure I had in my mind, and braved the waters of another country. I didn't have to go far. I boarded a train to Sweden on another sunny but cold Friday in March and set off to swim in the other side of the Øresund Strait 35 minutes away in Malmö, Sweden. I had walked along the white sand beach past Ribersborg Kallbadhus before, a traditional cold-water spa perched out in the sea between Denmark and Sweden, but I'd never actually been in. With a direct train ride from Copenhagen, it was a very easy place to start, or so I thought.

Kallis, as locals call it, is a Malmö institution. Built at the end of the nineteenth century, the open-air swimming bath had two open-water sea baths, five saunas and a hot tub, with views over the Øresund Strait across to Denmark. It had weathered its fair share of storms, survived two world wars, and had been rebuilt following fires and spring storms to become an icon of the city and much-beloved leisure facility. For just 70 Swedish kronor – around £5.40 – you can relax in the saunas, dip in the sea and bathe on the sundeck all afternoon if you want. They even do occasional midnight spas there, where you can bathe outside under the stars.

It sounded and seemed so utterly romantic and traditional that was the ideal place to start. There was one catch, though. I didn't realise until I'd walked through the turnstiles that it was a completely nude spa.

A door led to the sex-segregated changing rooms along a wooden slatted path. The same path led out to sea, with a saltwater pool on the right and sunbathing benches and platforms along the side. The view was to the sea, but all I noticed was that all the women were naked. I got changed in the changing rooms, hanging my clothes on a peg and stashing my bag under the wooden bench. Nearly every peg was festooned with winter coats, hats and scarves, and the lockers were almost full. I walked out, wrapped in a thin blue towel, and looked for a sign of what to do next. There was a small area with four showers, a corridor with rooms on the left and right, and a passageway leading outside to the sunny deck and the seawater pool. This was the women's section; to the left, an identical mirror image of this spa was open to men only.

At the back of the deck, a pathway led to wider wooden steps that went right down to the open sea. Women sat naked on towels in the sun, soaking up the Vitamin D through every pore of their bodies, with their eyes closed. By the showers, a sign on the wall said, 'Water temperature: 3.7°C. Air temperature: 5°C. Love Every Body.'

I stopped a large, heavily tattooed lady in her fifties and asked, a little helplessly: 'It's my first time here. What do I do?'

'Take a shower,' she said kindly. 'Then pick a sauna. There's a dry one, a wood-fired one, and a mixed one. Then swim in the sea, sunbathe, and do it all over again.'

So I showered and then, towel in hand, walked into the first door and opened it. My heart dropped like stone.

Packed into this small space, twelve men ranged up and down the three tiers of slatted wooden benches on one side, and about eight women on the side closest to me. Nobody's head swivelled as I walked in – they were all too busy talking – but it was the first time I'd been naked in mixed company amid strangers in public since I was about three years old, I reckoned, and it was absolutely typical that I would walk into the mixed sauna first. As if being naked in public wasn't bad enough, now I had to be naked in front of a bunch of men too. If the heat wasn't already bringing a flush to my cheeks, I would have been blushing furiously.

I took my seat quickly on the second tier on a little towel, trying not to look too awkward. A big picture window showed a wide-angle view of the sea, with rocks in the foreground and a far-off wind farm in the distance. I studied it. The sky was a perfect blue, the sea was more of a cobalt colour, and the granite rocks were splattered with lichen the colour of gorse flowers. Water hissed through a pipe onto the sauna oven in the corner and a cloud of steam rose.

Down and to the left of me, an older man with silver-grey hair had bubbles of sweat coming up on his back like liquid blisters. He was talking animatedly to the other men about football. I don't speak very good Swedish, but even I could understand the words 'Chelsea' and 'Abramovich'. Wherever you went in the world, someone was always talking about English football, it seemed.

I sat for longer, letting the football chat wash over me, noticing that the other women were all sitting quietly, zoning out, sweating. When the heat rising in my hair follicles was almost too hot to bear, I stood up and walked out into the cold hallway. The next step was to swim.

A confession: I hadn't ever swum naked in the sea before. I have friends who grew up by the sea for whom it was a rite of passage as a teenager to go skinny dipping at night, but there was not much cause for it where I grew up. In the Stockport of the 1990s, a greyish-brown arm of the River Mersey snaked its way through the town, littered with shopping trolleys and the twisted, rusting skeletons of old bikes. Skinny dipping there would have sent me straight to Stockport infirmary.

I walked down the steps and swam a few strokes. The sensation was completely different. I didn't feel like I was at a swimming pool, taking a swimming lesson or doing anything active or sporty at all.

Without the tug of Lycra straps on my shoulder and the containment of the costume around the top of my thighs and body, I felt free. I could sense all edges of my body in the same way, and it was like I was actually part of the water. It flowed around me, and my hair fanned out in the water. It supported me and surrounded me. It was glorious.

I was still me, of course, an awkward and not particularly confident English woman who has always found nudity a bit tricky. It's not in my nature to run around naked, and I'm not sure, even as a toddler, it ever was. I told myself that no one can see you when you're in the water, even in water as clear as this. It's my trick for getting round moments when I'd otherwise blush myself to death: just imagine that nobody can see you. While I was conjuring up a cloak of invisibility, the thought crossed my mind that if I hadn't left my job, I'd still be sitting in an office at this time of day, probably in a meeting that could have been an email. Instead, I was frolicking naked in the sea on a sunny day just because I felt like it. That felt just delicious: I was alive and full of energy and doing just what I wanted. I felt like myself.

I had a little pang of guilt as well: maybe I shouldn't really be having fun like this, like I had no cares and responsibilities in the world? Maybe I should be acting like everyone else and spending my life in the office and not in the sea. I was second guessing myself a bit. It's scary sometimes to admit that you want a different kind of life from the one that everyone else seems so happy with. I wasn't really sure I was allowed to do that, or allowed to think like that. A tiny part of me wondered if I was going to get caught out and told off for stepping outside the box. But looking around, it was obvious that I wasn't the only person finding this place joyful. Sure, there were a number of middle-aged and retired women lounging around, but there were younger women too, students, women in their twenties and thirties, with friends and on their own. I'm sure they hadn't all had a mid-career flip-out and burned their steady work lives to the ground: what were the chances? It just looked like they'd taken the morning off to do something that they enjoyed. Maybe they had flexible schedules; maybe they worked weekends and had two days off in the week? Maybe some worked 60 hours and were just snatching a single hour to recharge. There are so many different ways to live a life and to work, and it seemed likely that they were playing out in front of me. Perhaps, then, that's a kernel at the heart of creating a sustainable life you want to live: leaning into something a bit more flexible, and acknowledging that work doesn't have to be a straight 9–5 – and that the traditional paradigms don't suit everyone all the time. Having the freedom to find a tempo, pace and work life that suits you seems important – and there are other people out there making it happen.

In the water, in that moment, I felt healthy, integrated, a whole person, not just a replaceable cog in a wheel. I was writing my own story of bravery, relaxation and sinking into nature, all at the same time. I was just where I was supposed to be.

Within a minute or so, my toes were tingling and starting to go numb. It was a sign for me to come out, so I did. I dried off, sat in the sun for a few minutes, then showered off and headed to sauna number two.

There was a completely different feeling in the wood-fired sauna, a ladies-only sauna where a gentle ripple of Swedish chatter ran through it. I was relaxed already, and now concentrated on warming up my blotchy pink legs.

My eyes didn't stare so stonily out of the window this time, but glanced gently around the room. Two younger women tentatively came in, unsure about the nudity and about where to sit. They weren't Swedish either – maybe Portuguese? – and talked to each other uncertainly. They finally sat a little rigidly like I had in the last sauna, like they were on pins. An older woman stood up and walked out. She had glasses as thick as the end of a milk bottle on, and an almost institutional haircut, and as she walked out I could see a tattoo on her arm – a strong black women's lib symbol from the 1970s, a fist raised inside the graphic symbol for women. In that moment, I loved how much swimming could reveal of ourselves. You see unexpected tattoos telling stories of who you are on the inside, and who you were when you were younger too. There are stories written on our skin, stories under our skin and stories being written by our bodies at every turn.

I took my second naked sea swim in the open sea, not the seawater pool, stashing my towel and bottle of water in the wooden crate at the top of the steps. I pushed off the seaweedy bottom step into the clear blue water. Steam rose from the triangular shape of the ski slope cum power plant Copenhill in Copenhagen in the far distance.

The sea water was cold but invigorating. I wanted to stay in for longer. My skin tingled and I splashed the water on my face. I was still not brave enough to put my head under the water, but I was in for as long as I could bear, and then out and drying myself in the sunshine again.

I wrapped myself in a towel and sat in the sun on the deck. It was warm, much warmer than sun should be in early spring. The sea lapped gently at the steps and the wooden stilts the bathhouse was built on, and there wasn't a cloud in the sky. The sage-green buildings were in perfect harmony with the sea, the sun, the sky, the blonde sand dunes and the pale green sea grass, and everything felt good.

The final sauna was a silent sauna, a dry sauna, and it was packed. In one corner at the back, a woman read a paperback about the fall of Rome. Everyone else was sitting on the benches in a meditative atmosphere. A large wall poster in Swedish and English gave a rundown of the rules: always sit on a towel. Always dry off before you come in, otherwise you can lower the temperature of the sauna. No talking. No messing with the sauna equipment – that's for staff only. No body lotion or oils.

The picture window next to it was about the size of a small cinema screen and we were all riveted, watching the sea's gentle rise and fall. My cold toes started to come back to life. I felt completely relaxed. I dipped in the open sea one more time before I showered and layered up, ready for the cold outside. It seemed strange to pass people blanketed in scarves and huddled in thick winter coats as I walked across the wooden bridge and back to the sandy beach, when I'd spent the last hour and a half completely naked in and beside the sea.

As I cycled down the cobbled streets and back to the station, I could still feel the cold sea in my gloved fingers, and a stillness in my mind. According to the Kallis website, the endorphins produced by winter bathing last two to four hours, and they also improve mood and alleviate mild depression. 'When a winter swimmer exposes his body to the icy water,' it said, 'a firework is released by so-called endorphins, which are the body's own morphine. Many winter bathers emphasize that "the blood flows faster in the veins" after a dip.'

14

The plan was alive and well to swim around Scandinavia now I'd taken my first dips in Sweden. I still had a few plans to put together, but I already had Norway and Finland in my sights, and a little dream of swimming in the Arctic Sea, the coldest in the world, was on the horizon. It felt thrillingly challenging, and maybe a little too far beyond my comfort zone, but the idea of swimming at the top of the world seemed like the ultimate test of my cold-water swimming obsession. And as I worked on stories for newspapers and magazines about life in Scandinavia, I looked for a way to add a swim in wherever I was headed, and for swimmers I could meet when I was there.

I left a beautiful weekend filled with spring sunshine behind me and flew back into winter, headed for the Arctic Circle in Norway to write a feature about an unusual hotel. Denmark was experiencing early summer temperatures; people were lying out on the boardwalks along the harbour like cats in the sun. But instead of slathering on sun cream for my skin's first moment of contact with proper sun in six months, I layered up, pulling on my sheepskin-lined heavy duty winter boots and dug out my woolly gloves and ski underwear again.

As I landed in Bodø, a town 80 kilometres north of the Arctic Circle, I felt completely out of my depth. It was the furthest north in the world that I had ever been. Snow blew horizontally across the runway of the airport like sand in a sandstorm as we came into land. I thought about the flipflops and swimsuit I had packed in my suitcase. A full-blown blizzard chased me down the street as I tugged my roller suitcase through growing snowdrifts down to the ferry port. Tiny gritty snowflakes flew straight into my eyes, making lines of mascara run down my cheeks and settle in the wrinkles around my eyes.

A wild 40-minute boat ride took me to the island of Sørvær in the Fleinvær archipelago, a group of over 300 sparsely inhabited islands, and the location for an experimental hotel called the Arctic Hideaway, or, as a direct translation from its Norwegian name, the 'immersion room', a place where you can explore a deeper emotional relationship with nature and, by extension, yourself. This was where I was planning to take my first swim north of the Arctic Circle. I wasn't alone: running the hideaway were two caretakers, another Laura from Copenhagen, who also liked to winter bathe, along with her friend Jarl, and along for the ride were the hotel's multihyphenate founder/owner and jazz musician Håvard and his friend, Norwegian champion freediver Siri.

Every window of the common room and kitchen had a view of the water, along with the rough, ridged, low-lying islands that curved in the waves like the backs of whales. The higher ground was coloured moss green and there were browner traces of autumn die-back grass at lower levels. As the ferry crested the corner of the island and came in to dock, a great sea eagle with a vast wingspan swooped by in greeting, as if to say: *You're in the wilds now. In this place, nature is in charge.*

Later that afternoon, as I watched from the wall-to-wall window in the lounge, a small tern battled the wind in the bay, like a salmon swimming upstream. It nudged forward inch by inch, its determination undimmed by the power of the wind. *Maybe I'm that small seabird too,* I thought, *imagining I could swim in a place like this that's made for majestic sea eagles, not small fry like me. Perhaps I should be leaving it all to people more connected to this kind of scenery, the Norwegians and the Danes.*

I wrapped up in all my warmest clothes and took a wander out along the rocky shoreline, by banks of floating bladderwrack and seaweed-covered rocks to see if I could spot the shy sea otters who lived there. All I found were some discarded scallop shells, the remains of their dinner. The rain washed the windows and a lonely chair, angled for maximum sun, sat against the fish-scale-tiled kitchen building outside. I could see, in my mind's eye, how this place would look in the sun on a bright day, how turquoise the water would be, how blue the sky. But today the water looked flinty and wind-chased, racing and restless. I felt the solidity of the rock the hotel was built on, as the water carried on its harried pace around it. The sky dimmed and darkened, and more rain came in. The outer edges of my worries washed away, sand-blown and contextualised by the wildness of the nature around me. In the moment, in this wild place, life felt real. You could breathe it, and feel it. The harried thoughts in my mind calmed down. There was only one thing in charge in this remote place and that was nature. Beside the power of the wind and the depth of the sea here, I was nothing. I was small in the great scheme of things, and that smallness felt comforting. I didn't have to do it all, be it all, hold it all together. I could trust that things were unfolding just as they were supposed to.

Building a hotel on an island like this takes a certain type of person. Håvard, the hideaway's owner, is unique, a champion of quiet voices and quiet places, but simultaneously a wild spirit himself, with a punchy personality and an unwavering belief in the value of nature to culture and life itself. It was his idea to build a space in a remote place to accommodate creatives looking for something different, and to offer it as a hotel for those willing to travel off the beaten track to find a wilder side to their soul. It's an immersive experience, and something that deepens day after day in this quiet but enormously dramatic place, where the weather changes by the minute, winds shift, clouds blow, and the glowering mountains of Arctic Norway look on, sometimes hidden by clouds, sometimes framing every view.

In the few days I spent there, the sea consumed me. I spent hours staring out of the window watching the sea change colour and the clouds gather and pass overhead. It was the background noise and the soundtrack to everything. Its changing colour fascinated me, showing Caribbean blue in the sandy bays of the island, and a deeper navy where the channel sank to its deepest spot. There was no rhythm to the day beyond the sun rising and setting, and the short winter day in between. There was nothing to do but immerse yourself in nature, read books about whales and seaweed, bake cakes and bread in the kitchen, and take walks in the freezing cold air, where taking my hands out of their gloves to take a photo with my phone turned my skin a livid pink.

In the afternoons, Jarl started the sauna, giving us a place to gather and commune. A dark wooden cave with only a small window set on the old ferry-boat pier, a couple of metres over the water, it filled rapidly with the scent of pine. The window misted and the omnipresent sound of the sea was replaced with the hiss of steam. We chatted about Norway and Denmark, and the differences between the two, comparing old grievances like families at Christmas. Jarl added an empty beer can to the collection on the small windowsill as time went on, further dimming the light.

At nearly 100 degrees, we jointly agreed that it was too hot to bear, and piled out into the wind and cold, walking along the frozen path to the other ferry platform, which had a ladder to the clear blue sea. My flipflops got an outing on the ice-edged path; as I looked down to the shoreline, even the rock pools by the sea edge had iced over. Jarl hurled himself in from the top, splashing us all over; I climbed down the ladder with Laura and swam, breath catching in the cold, frigid toes and fingers seemingly freezing on contact with the water. I had the taste of salt on my lips. The walk back to the sauna was brisk and joy filled, and we repeated it again and again.

The next day, I climbed to the highest point in the archipelago, a hill behind the hotel. The clouds had lifted and huge mountains loomed into view, their dark brown craggy faces decorated with snow, like a chocolate cake dusted with icing sugar. I wanted so desperately to see the family of orca that Laura had seen a few days earlier, hunting in the sound, but there was nothing there but views of the sea. In the direction I was looking, the next piece of land was the east coast of Greenland, complete with its local swimmers: polar bears.

We fired up the sauna again in the afternoon, and Jarl, Siri and I sat in it, warming through, and going to swim when it got too hot. My second Arctic swim felt better than the first – despite this being the Arctic Ocean, the temperature was around 4°C, broadly similar to Copenhagen harbour, thought far saltier. I even dipped my head under and floated happily for a few moments before climbing back up the ladder.

But as I walked back to the sauna things started to feel a little strange. While the air temperature was -1°C, the wind chill made it feel like -8°C. It was like tiny needles were pressing into my flesh. My pink legs were spotted with white dots. Back in the dark wooden box of the sauna, the heat was higher than ever. Jarl added logs and water to the oven. I didn't feel right.

I sat for a few moments trying to figure out what I was feeling. The room was hot, I knew it was hot, but my body felt cold. I felt like I was covered with frog skin – my clammy skin was cold to the touch, slimy with sweat, but I was sitting in a very hot room. It was as if my head and body weren't communicating with each other.

Håvard started to talk to me, congratulating me on swimming in the Arctic Ocean, but I batted him away. I grunted no to a beer. I stepped out of the sauna, resting against the wall in the wind, feeling colder and colder. Then I grabbed my clothes and headed for the shower. I washed quickly under a hot shower and threw on my clothes, first the ski underwear on top and bottom, then my jeans, T-shirt and heat tech jumper. I walked quickly back to my cabin and huddled up under the duvet.

Ten minutes later, there was a semi-naked man at the window – Jarl – in his shorts in the cold wind, checking I was OK. I gave him a thumbs up and felt guilty about running out on them without saying anything. But my body just did what it had to do, there had been very little thinking involved.

I sank back under the duvet and gave in to what my body needed: sleep and warmth. I was physically overwhelmed.

Things improved as the evening came. Ole, an old friend of Håvard's, was visiting from the Lofoten Islands, and brought some fermented air-dried fish for dinner. We sat and ate and talked, and I picked the bones from my teeth as delicately as I could. Håvard concocted an unusual hot chocolate with a dash of chartreuse liqueur as an after-dinner treat, and we sat on sheepskin-clad stools around the table watching YouTube videos of Norwegian jazz.

One by one, we started yawning and getting ourselves dressed in multiple layers to go the ten metres back down the path to our cabins in the dark, but we were stopped in our tracks by the sheer force of nature. In the night sky, the northern lights were breaking into soft-edged lines and graceful flourishes, flaming against the dark sky. Everyone else gradually went to bed, but I still sat there watching as they formed and reformed, chasing the stars across the sky. It was one of the most beautiful things I've ever seen.

I returned to the mainland during another snowstorm and I went for a meeting in the chic café in the local library. Through the window I could see Pust, the sauna I'd booked to visit in the afternoon, a floating platform with wooden struts arranged on it reminiscent of the big wooden fish-drying racks used in this part of Norway, or, if you've never seen them, like a giant wooden clothes airer. The snow slowly started to clear and the sun came out; the sea was grey-blue.

While swimming on Sorvær was a singular experience, for its cut-off, nature-encircled island vibe, swimming in Bodø had some significance too. This town is not just the biggest cultural centre in this part of northern Norway, it's also the location of the strongest tidal current in the world, the Saltstraumen, a churning stretch of water beset with changing, twisting pockets of water. Whirlpools of up to ten metres across and five metres down are created when vast amounts of water whip through the narrow passage between the Saltenfjord and Skjerstadfjord. Three thousand cubic metres of water are driven through this channel every second, and the sea rises and falls by a depth of two metres here twice a day. This pressure and unique topography make the twisting pockets of water form, pulling fish and floating masses of seaweed and kelp in and out of the channel, and driving water down to the depths. When you think of a classical whirlpool, something you might see depicted in a gilt-framed oil painting in a national art gallery, you have a sense of the power that these things have. At Saltstraumen, there are so many whirlpools you can't even count them.

Overseen by a tall grey bridge, there's an island in the middle of the stretch of water, 412 metres at its narrowest, and a wild series of churning, changing, twisting pockets of water all the way along. In *Waterlog*, Roger Deakin's wonderful book about swimming Great Britain, his great unrealised ambition is to swim across the Corryvreckan whirlpool in Scotland, the unnavigable third-largest whirlpool in the world. There's a woman in Bodø who has swum the Saltstraumen, not once, but twice. It doesn't feel like a swimming journey of Scandinavia without a mention of her record-breaking swim.

Dagmar Dahl isn't your average swimmer. Not only has she been swimming since the age of two, she's also an Associate Professor of Sports at Nord University in Bodø, and is a swimming and lifesaving instructor. She's warm and passionate, and runs her own cold-water swimming group in Bodø called The Penguins, where she regularly sees swimmers undergo the exact transformation I've been going through, growing stronger and developing more self-esteem and confidence as they do.

At the age of 50, she became the first Norwegian to swim the Saltstraumen, joining an ultra-elite group of six people in the world to ever do so. And it was far from an easy task: swimming across this dangerous stretch of water takes guts and belief, training and precision timing. You have to check the tide table and the phases of the moon to catch the calmest and least dangerous moment to swim the strait, the sweet spot being the exact point between the full and new moon, when the difference between the tides is lowest and the stream is the weakest. At either end – when the moon is full or at the new moon point – the stream and tide are at their strongest.

And then, at this precise point, you have to swim in a short time window when the tide is turning. Precision timing and training are important – this is a dangerous operation in every direction. Dagmar trained so she would be able to withstand the 11-degree water for up to 40 minutes, and had an experienced RIB captain in his boat beside her. She took a route near the island with the boat beside her, so in the worst-case scenario, she would drift out to sea and he could pick her up. If you swim too far inland, away from the island and the bridge, she explained, you can be sucked down under the surface.

'When I first saw the Saltstraumen, I was fascinated by the phenomenon,' she told me. 'It's so beautiful there. I just thought it would be amazing to swim it.'

Dagmar first swam the Saltstraumen on 12 July 2020, during the turning tide, and then a month later, on 28 August.

'The first time, I got caught by the stream when I passed the island in the middle,' she said. 'I tried to swim in a straight line and then I tried to adjust my course, but I had to accept the tide was stronger than me. It was calmer in the middle, but then I caught the next edge. I wasn't panicking but I was fighting it hard. I had to drift more and had to accept that it would take me a little under the bridge, drifting to the bay by the lifesaving buoy. It was funny to see the swim on the GPS after. I was shocked to see that I had swum over 600 metres.

'The second time was better. It was a grey and rainy morning. It was unpredictable but a bit calmer in the water than the first time. I was a bit more nervous because I knew what could happen, but then again I was there to enjoy it – it wasn't a new world record this time. I stood and watched it for a long time before I went in – I was so impressed, it was so beautiful with so many jellyfish and algae floating in it. It was amazing.

'As I swam past the island, the sun came out. If you are not religious, that is the kind of experience that is enough to make you believe! I swam the last 25 metres butterfly. It was so fantastic! To cap off the whole experience, when I got back to the boat, two porpoises started to swim alongside it.'

Two years after the event, joy, delight and pride filled her voice as she recounted her adventures. It is an extraordinary achievement and a terrifically daring act of swimming overall. I fell in love with her passion and her impromptu decision, to think that on seeing a stretch of churning water, she wanted to swim it. There's something really special about Dagmar's story too, something empowering and spiritual. She's not there to fight nature and prove her dominion over it; she's there to respect and observe it, to cherish it and to marvel at its raw power. And just for a few moments, to be part of it.

The images of her swimming as the sun came out, and of dolphins following her boat, lingered in my head for days afterwards.

Relaxing in Pust floating sauna later in Bodø, I watched the weather turn from sunny with blue skies to snow flurries with blue skies. Big boats and little boats lined the marina where we swam; only metres away the large island ferries docked. A slick snake of oil gleamed in a few places in the dark water. In the near distance, around the edge of a spit of land, a camouflaged military boat sneaked along, as invisibly as it could. Military exercises had ramped up in recent days in the north of Norway, where the border with Russia was not so far away.

In the sauna, a middle-aged blonde lady wearing a strawberry-red swimsuit added some citrus oil to the water bowl and tossed it on the oven. It hissed and the air filled with the scent of summer in Italy. Over the course of the hour, we swam three times from the ladder at one end of the platform to the next one, perhaps fifteen metres along in the harbour, breathing little clouds from our mouths as we did.

Snow started to gently fall, lighting on the water and vanishing, while impenetrable grey clouds blocked the colour from the sky and the tops of the nearby islands from view. Snow fell on the path outside the sauna, disguising the ice on the path I walked with naked feet. Unlike the others, I didn't have neoprene socks on. For the first few steps, I noticed it, but then numbness took over. This was the coldest sea I'd ever swum in, I had no doubt about that, and I'd stayed in the water for longer here than I had anywhere else. I felt like I'd smashed the challenge of swimming in the Arctic and it hadn't been as hard as I'd thought. I was inspired and excited about what might come next. I wondered what it would feel like to swim back in Copenhagen harbour after experiencing the wilds of Norway.

15

Back in Denmark, as the mid-point of April came and went, it was like someone had switched on a light. The wind was still wintry, but the sun shone long and hard, all morning and all evening, and the kids came home from school with red faces from spending so much time playing outside in the wind. In the morning in the harbour, the tide was in and the air suddenly smelt of brine and seaweed. When I walked the dog up the hill, blossom had burst all over the trees and the birds surprised me with how loudly they sang. Spring was here, and it didn't care who knew.

At a new swimming spot, Hanna and I were swimming two or three times a week, and really swimming now. We swam out to the buoys and back, like swimming the width of a swimming pool, not just for a few strokes in the freezing water. We liked it so much that we got out of the water and then got in again, swimming twice. The second time always felt more delicious, less cold, more enjoyable. The water was around us and part of us and we floated with the tide. Soon, I was diving off the wooden side, a metre above the water, down to the green depths, coming up and brushing my wet hair out of my eyes completely refreshed. It was still cold, but it didn't matter. After the challenge of winter, the dare to ourselves to swim in cold water and the physical test of it all, the spring brought something else: fun.

Towards the end of the month, long-legged benches started cropping up in prominent places around the city. They looked like normal iron city benches, but on stilts, as if a growing potion had been painted just on their legs and they'd extended overnight. In all other respects, the benches were just the same. In the town hall square, tourists climbed up and sat on the top for selfies. I wondered if they spotted the plaque at the back that said what they were all about.

TV2, our local TV station, had got together with the city authorities and created these eye-catching leggy benches as a stark reminder about climate change. The idea was that they showed what the rising water temperatures were going to do to the city by 2100 physically, rather than try to tell people with facts and statistics. It's not just that we would need to raise the legs of the benches to be able to sit comfortably without getting wet, it's that we would all need to be able to swim that gets me. In a city built across a series of islands, wherever you are in the old town or tourist centre, you've likely got a view of the water. I watch the water in the evenings as I'm writing, the streetlights reflected in it as the sun goes down. By 2100 my first-floor flat would be OK if the sea level rose by this much, but the ground floor flat below us would be flooded up to the ceiling. I'll probably be able to dive in from my balcony.

My trip to Norway had done nothing to dim my lust for adventure. In fact, completely the opposite. I cancelled our family holiday to Italy and announced around the kitchen table one night that we would just have to go back to this incredible hotel. I couldn't bear the thought that I'd been to such an extraordinary place in the world and my husband and kids hadn't. They protested at how they wanted to eat real Italian food and sit in the sunshine, but I would not be moved: we were going and if they liked it even a tiny bit as much as I had, it would be fuel for their souls.

I wrote my story about Håvard's hotel in the middle of nowhere and filed it with my editor, and I felt a great sense of accomplishment. It wasn't about the writing, but about the fact that I'd found a way to wrap the writing, the adventure and the swimming together. Those three things that I'd said I wanted to base my year on – being creative, swimming and meeting new people – were actually coming together. Where I'd been steering the ship away from what I knew I didn't like, I was now steering it actively towards something. The time and space I'd been able to carve out had at least given me the chance to figure out the direction I wanted to go in. I wondered if maybe that was the key to a good life. I dropped my hours in my part-time job and started taking on a few more writing projects that made sense instead.

It felt uncommonly good to be free of an office but able to work and participate in other people's projects. And even at my part-time job, swimming had a small role. We started a swim group in the office, meeting before work to dip in the harbour together before cycling on to a hot coffee at work.

What if this was really all there was to living a good life: decide the three things you want to do, which bring you the most joy, and just do them, repeatedly? I know it sounds deceptively simple, but maybe it is? It doesn't have to be a dramatic change: you don't have to flounce out of the office like a diva, which, looking back, I feel I had. You could just integrate these ideas: what if I swim once a week? What if I make an effort to meet someone new every month? What if I do something creative at the weekend? And it doesn't have to be those things – it's just an example. On my return from Norway, I was feeling like this could be one of the keys that unlocks a good life, for me, and maybe, just maybe, I'd found a way to make it work.

Denmark's premier mermaid, Karin Lund Madsen, was a ray of sunshine on a grey and windswept day, standing beside a snack stand at Svanemøllen beach. She gave me a big grin and an even bigger hug and we started off down the sand, chatting nineteen to the dozen. She hefted her large silicon tail over her shoulder and laid it down where the water reached the sand. As I started to peel off my layers and she took off her rainbow-striped hand-knitted jumper and wrapped a flimsily decorated lace bikini top around her, she filled me in on her journey so far from being an actor in a children's theatre to working as the mermaid in the national aquarium.

'I was inspired by the Weeki Wachee mermaids in Florida,' she said, her long brown hair blowing in the breeze. This troupe of mermaids are based in Florida at Weeki Wachee Springs and have been performing for the public since 1947 in a theatre twenty feet underwater. Water pipes, which they sip, feed them with oxygen so they can stay underwater for longer, dancing and waving and performing, eating and drinking, for anyone who wants to see them in their underwater space. A visit to these natural springs got Karin thinking about what it would be like to bring a mermaid show to Denmark. She now regularly performs for children in a tank full of sharks at the weekend and on school holidays, and puts on shows and displays in various towns around the Danish coast.

As we started to strike out into the sea, Karin up to her waist in an orange-gold silicone rubber tail which meant she had to shuffle and then crawl into the gradually deepening sea, she told me how she ended up at the Danish National Aquarium, Den Blå Planet, when she was pregnant with her first child.

'I'm a fish nerd,' she said. 'And just as they were developing the new aquarium, they needed someone like me.'

With experience and education in fish keeping, plus a certain creative, wacky spirit, she helped develop the storytelling, theatre and marketing of the new aquarium, which is the biggest in Northern Europe. Before long, she decided that watching the fish in the tank wasn't enough: she wanted to join them.

What Karin has created is unique in Denmark – she dives underwater, holds her breath for up to 1 minute and 40 seconds, and performs, interacting with the public and the fish in the largest tank in the aquarium. She also holds shows in other locations around Denmark, diving in the sea, showing off her tail and waving to a disbelieving public. It's quite an accomplishment in the land of *The Little Mermaid* to be the national mermaid.

She doesn't do it alone either – she has a troupe of other mermaids to call on too, most of whom are former freedivers. She's found that it's easier to teach a freediver to act than teach an actor to dive, the only issues being that you have to find ways to encourage them to let go of their competitive instinct so they can embrace it properly.

water was deep and cold out at the edge of the beach, where the walkway reached out and the shores of Sweden glimmered in the distance. Fronds of seaweed and long leaves of seagrass brushed my feet as we really started to swim, chatting and swapping stories about our shared love of swimming. And then for the dive. We breathed in, counting down slowly from three, and then ducked under and went as deep as possible. Karin was a metre below me, practised and comfortable in the depths. I wanted to go deeper too but it was like that part of the watery world was shut off from me: my lungs were pulling me up and everything, including my legs, felt too light to get to the same depth. I watched from the middle of the water instead. The haze of the blue-green water makes it look like a dream, swimming with a mermaid, her tail rippling beneath the sea. All too quickly, my lungs were bursting and I had to come up for air.

We chatted some more and then dove down again, this time not so deep and for not quite so long. Karin was a long way beneath me this time, and I reached out with my arms, trying to pull myself further under the water, but it just made me aware that I was not at home this far under water and maybe never would be. I couldn't see the bottom, just rippling deep green shapes and the struts of the pier standing out against the green. Karin's long brown hair flowed out behind her. I tried again to go deeper, to get into this underwater underworld with her. Being surrounded head to toe by utterly cold water was intoxicating; swimming in the same space as her made me realise how far there was to go in this swimming journey. I might have been happy in the cold water now, but there were greater depths to plumb. But then brain freeze gripped me like a vice and I swam up to the surface. Then Karin surfaced too, also with brain freeze, and I didn't feel quite so inadequate.

We swam back to the shallows, surfacing on the sandy beach. Shivering took over, followed by an adrenaline rush. Staying in the water that long had clearly given my system a bit of a boost. Maybe going all in, going underwater, even to the shallow depths that I did, was the solution to finding that rush again. Wrapped up in jumpers again, we sat at the snack hut with our hands encircling paper cups of hot chocolate. She put her tail in a red waterproof holdall with 'Air Greenland' written across it in white letters.

'You've been to Greenland?' I said. 'Tell me more.'

Between shivers and sips of hot chocolate, she talked about sailing from the port, not far from here in northern Copenhagen, through the night and on into the darkness across the North Atlantic, waking up to the sight of the glittering white icebergs of Greenland. I thought about my dream of swimming there, if I was brave enough, sometime in the future.

Hot chocolates drained, we sat and talked until I'd curled my cardboard cup up into a cone and then a strange origami shape, and the plastic and paper had started to pull away from each other. It was time for Karin to pick her baby up for a playdate with a friend, and for me to get home and get back to some work.

'This isn't the last time we'll swim together, is it?' she said, as she gave me a hug goodbye.

'Definitely not,' I replied, and promised to come see her swim at the aquarium sometime.

Meeting new people: tick. Doing something creative: tick. Swimming: tick. It was coming together. I was still shivering from the cold on my cycle home along the waterfront, but I was smiling all the way.

Sometimes you don't have to leave your country to have an adventure. Sometimes it's just a case of finding one on your doorstep.

As we got into May, I realised that I hadn't had a cold or been sick since I started this winter bathing plan. It didn't feel possible: I used to get regular colds and would catch everything going, any bug, sniffle or cough that the kids and their friends could bring home with them. Of course, as soon as I realised this, I started to feel a bit off key.

Feeling too tired to swim, and a bit too tired to commit myself to the work I had planned to do, I decided to do something good for myself anyway, and took my dog for a long walk up our nearest green hill in the morning instead. We walked past a hedge full of chirping sparrows and up to a path lined with dandelions which, in this early part of the season, looked like bright wildflowers. Max ran grinning along the top of the hill, his ears flapping, then we took a path through an arching tunnel of white cherry blossom and five-petalled hawthorn flowers like stars back down along the water.

I stood and watched it flow from the bridge over the sluice. It was flowing on and on into the city, past the little red fishermen's huts towards the twisted towers and ancient architecture of the city and out to sea. A pair of cormorants dipped their necks sinuously in and out of the water. Two girls in their twenties wrangled with a bright green kayak, pushing it off from the side of the canal with their black plastic paddles.

I stood and took it all in, all the blue, all the currents, all the life of the water and the harbour in front of me. I was part of it in my own small way: I was part of something, for once, and I felt like I belonged. There was something like hope in the air. I wondered if there was anything more life affirming than deciding that you want to do something, doing it, and seeing it work out. If you could go swimming with a mermaid on a cold day in Denmark, you could do anything, right?

16

The city's annual harbour clean hit the headlines in the local newspaper, and this year, the municipality's divers didn't just find a hundred-and-one old bikes, seven shopping trolleys and a little less rubbish than in previous years, but two rifles as well. They had been handed over to the police, the news report said, with a shocked air as if it was impossible to imagine anyone sinking weapons into the water at night. With a city harbour this size, and the diversity of people living along it, it didn't surprise or shock me at all. After all, Nordic Noir had been a cultural fixture for years. Crime dramas starring grumpy male detectives and their quirky or troubled but beautiful female counterparts have been one of the city's biggest exports for years. The contrast between the drama shown on the telly and my experiences of being in the city, which feels safe to me at all times of day or night, is strong. But that said, on the day we moved into our harbourside apartment, a police diver brought up a sawn-off shotgun in the water right outside our window. Copenhagen is a super-safe place to live, but there are criminal elements everywhere.

Despite it being cleaner, as the water temperature started to creep up and the wind started to die back, just a little, I was finding it harder and harder to swim. I was making a point of going swimming twice a week at least, but it suddenly felt much more of a chore than it had before. Perhaps all the time in floating saunas in the earlier part of the year had caused a problem. I could easily face an hour of hot and cold therapy, but a morning with just a cold dip felt too hard. It was as if my body couldn't face it anymore, as if it had run out of energy and appetite for the cold. But I still wasn't going to quit. It was a deal I'd made to myself and I wanted to see it through. I gritted my teeth and bore it, stripping down to my swimsuit quickly on the cold dock, climbing down the ladder and into the water, swimming and swimming and swimming. Across the water on the Sluseholmen side, a woman jumped off a houseboat and swam for a long time, around the houseboats and across the water to the bright orange ladder, where she trod water for a few minutes before climbing out. She looked serene, unconcerned. I wanted to emulate her and her long swim, marvelling that she could be in there for so long at this temperature.

The next morning was sunny and the sea was as calm as a millpond. We dipped in a new corner of the harbour, cordoned off with yellow buoys from the rest of the traffic, and swam in clear water beside tiny translucent jellyfish.

There's a zen expression that says the way you do one thing is the way you do everything. I started wondering if that was true of swimmers too – is the way you swim the way you do everything? Or is the way you do everything reflected somehow in how you swim?

One of my friends, Kasia, just dips. Down the ladder and in the water, then up the ladder again. No swimming, just a dunk in the water, holding on to the ladder and out. It's the same every time. Even after a sauna by the water: in and out. She knows what she wants and she does it. She isn't pressured by what anyone else is doing. She just does things her way, meeting the challenge head on and getting what she wants from it. I'm not judging her. Well, not much. It's not like I'm staying in the water for half an hour in the biting cold and trying to win a record for how much I can take. I know that everyone has their habits and ideas about this cold-water swimming thing and, honestly, that's what makes it fun! It makes me curious, though. Her body must be accustomed to the cold by now. Why doesn't she want to swim too?

Sonia swims with finesse. Grace and beauty are the watchwords here: when she goes in the water, you can pick up a tiny bit in her movements that it's cold and she doesn't truly want to do it, but she hides it really well in her calm face and broad gestures. On the surface, everything is perfection. The only indication that she is swimming in the single-figure degree harbour water in a city in Northern Europe, rather than in a temperate Instagram-perfect infinity pool in the Indian Ocean, is when she gets out and immediately bursts into a wide grin. Her swan-like serenity masks the shock of the cold really well.

Hanna climbs down the ladder in a no-nonsense style and strikes out for the buoys. She's always the first to call a swim session and she rarely cries off. She is the instigator of all of our sessions and the one who pushes us to do more, to get out and swim again, to swim on a snowy day, to just keep swimming. She swims fast and confidently, with a clear direction. I have only seen her once dither on the steps in around 30 swims together, all through the winter. She's got a clarity and direction that just has to be admired, and from what I know about her outside the water, it's true. If you want to get something done, she's the one you ask.

And me? I'm an instigator too, in swimming as in life. I like to push boundaries and I'm always interested in trying something new. I'm creative and I'll try anything. I am the one who started the idea of swimming to the buoys and back. I will follow and match anything Hanna suggests. I don't want to be left behind. I'll rarely cry off, and I'll always try to swim the furthest, push the most: I'm not satisfied otherwise. My absolute favourite thing is to dive from the top of the deck down into the dark, cold green water.

I'm not completely fearless – far from it. I just decided that I don't want to let fear stop me. I have to gear up to these things – to the diving, for example – but sometimes I deliberately underprepare because I am afraid that thinking about it too much will stop me from doing it. I look the challenge in the face and do it. I just don't look too deeply, because that would scare me.

I spent so much time in the office overthinking and getting in my head about things that this feels like a relief to find a better balance between my body and mind. I have this powerful physical feeling, a gut feeling, that the life I'm trying to lead is the right thing to do, and that gut feeling is pulling me along. The diving in, the swimming, all of this is part of a wake-up call for my body: it's just as important as my brain. I'm enjoying getting to know it again.

I also feel like throwing myself headlong into this new life is the way to make it work. Dipping a toe in, at this point, when I've marked out a year to discover what makes me happy and how I can live better in the world, feels like it's not enough. There's a need to make the most of this pause, to make it count. I want to swing big because I think it will be rewarded; what is gained from playing small? I would feel sheepish and defeated if I didn't give it enough effort, and ended up in an office somewhere just going through the motions this time next year. If I've given it as much effort as I can, ending up there would be fine, but not if I haven't really tried. So sure, I'm diving in.

I don't dive gracefully but I'm hopeful that with more practice, I might one day. And unlike Sonia, you can tell from looking at my face exactly what I'm thinking.

It was not just about the swimming; it was about everything. Because for me it was true: the way you do one thing is the way you do everything.

As the month went on, work became more hectic and I started to feel that familiar burnout flicker on the edge of my vision. I was doing too much, without much focus, running from one thing to another in a pattern I recognised all too well. I was too busy to swim with the usual gang one week and I noticed the difference in my body and mind. I was jumpier, frustrated, hemmed in. I needed to stretch out and reclaim myself and my place in nature.

Missing the group swim, I arm-twisted my oldest daughter into swimming with me on a sunny afternoon in bone-cold water. The harbour was now coming alive with speedboats, pleasure boats and floating platforms chugging up and down the busy corridors. To my surprise, after multiple feints and toe dips, she actually did it, going down the slippery seaweedy ladder to her waist, waiting a beat, and then coming back up. Good for her. She was beaming and could now say she was part of the club. She described it perfectly too. 'It's like eating an extra strong mint,' she said. 'But you can feel it all over your body.' Seeing her bravery grow made me feel proud. Swimming with her made it fun again, and suddenly, the malaise of the last few weeks had dissolved and

I was back on track and loving it again. It reminded me how important it was to try new things and open up new worlds, to other people as well as myself. You never know where they might take you.

Norway called again, and I couldn't say no. Mid-month, I finally made it to Oslo to swim in the fjord and meet Siri Østvold, the freediver I met at the Arctic Hideaway back in March. I'd swum in Bergen and in Bodø, but I'd never even been to Oslo, let alone swum there. I scanned the tourist board website looking for urban swim spots, and booked into a hotel with the word 'sea' in its name, just because it seemed like a good omen.

I walked the streets from my hotel along row after row of boats in the marina, all the way to the dancing lines of the opera house and the Sørenga Sjøbad seawater pool. It was right at the end of the harbour, looking out to the fjord and its islands, with what appeared to be an industrial shipping container park not as far away as I would have liked on one side. Across the expanse of water and the harbour, I could see the swoop of the Holmenkollen ski jump in the hills beyond the city. The seawater pool had a serious dose of Nordic style to it – clean and minimalist, its wooden decking had sharp lines and enclosed a couple of swimming areas, with lanes marked out and ladders at each end. Another ladder led down to the open fjord from another part of the wooden decking, and benches stood around for people to rest on, along with a couple of open public shower points in the middle of the deck.

On a sunny weekend day, it would be thronging with people sunbathing, posing and swimming splashy lengths of front crawl in the four-lane pool. It was protected from the rougher water of the harbour by a floating deck in a way that reminded me of the iconic Icebergs pool in Bondi, Sydney. On any other day of the week, it probably would be thronging with people too, all colour and sound and one too many speaker systems pumping out Nordic electro into the air. Knowing Scandinavia, it would probably involve a little public nudity too. But none of that was in view today. I was there on the morning after Norway's big party, its national constitution day, when the country celebrates until long into the night. It was all but deserted.

A pair of construction workers ate snacks on their morning break, a tourist prowled with a large camera in hand, and a class of kindergarten kids played on the man-made beach beside the pool. In the emerald-green water, there was barely a ripple. Four long, cool lanes stretched out before me. I changed quickly and climbed in, surprised at how warm it felt compared to Copenhagen. There was very little debris of any type floating in the water or growing on the steps or up the wood: no seaweed, no jellyfish, just clear water and lots of it. It was lovely to swim in, but something was different and I couldn't put my finger on it. The salt stung my skin a little as I swam breaststroke up and down the lanes leaving a little ripple behind me. All was calm. I felt like I had the place all to myself, and honestly, if I was going to create my own private swimming pool, I could have done a lot worse.

Across the deck, the Oslo fjord beckoned. A sailboat moved past a small wooded island. The hulking shape of the DFDS ferry stood at dock like a bad mood. I walked across the platform and slipped down into the fjord, trying it on for size. It felt deep and unfettered, unlimited somehow, in a way I didn't quite like after the containment of the swim lane in the protected pool. It too was devoid of seaweed; nearby, a Seabin swirled the water around like a mini whirlpool and sucked plastic and debris down into its bucket. It skimmed the water, intercepting floating microplastics and litter, cleaning the water in the process.

It was a perfect day for swimming: the sky was blue, there was barely a breeze and I swam without hesitation, feeling the water surround me and support me. I wondered if I should swim out to the buoys floating a hundred metres out in the harbour, but instead decided to float, tread water, and soak up the atmosphere of this new swimming spot. I swam a little more and then got out, showering and then sitting wrapped in a towel on a bench looking out to the fjord. A little further down the waterfront, a long trailing line of cherry blossom petals blew into the moving water of the main harbour area.

I prised Siri from her work mid-afternoon for a coffee and a chat. A long-limbed sylph of a woman, blonde, poised and considered, she wouldn't be out of place in a James Bond film, perhaps diving for clams or fishing with a spear. I had a feeling her swimming style would be quite different from mine.

Siri is as at home in the water as she is on land. She took up freediving in 2019 and very quickly ascended to glory. She was the reigning Norwegian champion in no fins freediving, and could happily swim 60 metres or more beneath the surface without a mask or flippers, at home in a world that most of us will only ever see on wildlife documentaries. As we sat chatting by the window of a bakery in central Copenhagen, she spotted the Crown Prince and Princess of Norway wandering by. They looked just like any other couple their age, walking happily together around the city, except for the too-buff-for-his-navy-blue-suit bodyguard walking a few metres behind them, his finger glued to a transparent earpiece. First the mermaid, now the princess. I had that feeling, like I had in the Swedish woods, that there's something inescapably fairytale-like about living in this part of the world.

Like many of the swimmers I'd met, Siri's great love of water was born when she was a child. Growing up just outside Oslo, her parents sailed, so she was around water since she was a baby. She got her first snorkel mask at the age of four, and her family nicknamed her 'the seal' because they just couldn't get her out of the water. Before getting into freediving, she was surfing, snorkelling and pursuing all kinds of water sports as a hobby. The thing that really hooked her on the freediving was the transcendental feeling that it inspired in her.

'It's a pursuit where you look inwards, not outwards,' she said. 'As soon as I started doing it, I felt – now I'm home. It just felt natural. It did something to me that I didn't expect.'.

This instinctive pull to get right under the waves instead of surf on top of them led Siri to join Oslo's freediving club, and then to crush records in freediving for Norway. Not only can she dive to more than 60 metres below the ocean's surface, but she's also dived with humpback whales, sharks and orca, the latter in the Arctic north of Norway.

'I had this feeling that they knew I was there,' she said. Her face lit up as she told me all about the experience of swimming with an orca, close to a fishing boat, near the Lofoten Islands in Norway. Not only did she get into the water at the first available moment, but she stayed under the water, watching the great cetacean as it slowly swam round and turned to face her when she did so. She felt a great connection with this huge creature, meeting it in its own habitat.

Unlike a normal person, the thought of being face to face with one of these gigantic killing machines didn't phase her: super knowledgeable about the ocean, she decided that they were too clever to hurt her. Orca have been known to slice apart sharks and pinpoint just their livers to eat, and she knew that if they'd wanted to, they could do that to her. But she trusted that they wouldn't.

Rain started splashing the Oslo cobbles and when it became clear that it wasn't going to stop, we ordered more coffee and settled in for the afternoon. Swimming was off this afternoon, but I had a question only a local swimmer could answer. I asked Siri whether there was an app or way of monitoring if the water in the harbour was safe to swim in. After all, I'd just jumped in this morning, but I had seen a huge cruise ship and industrial works along the water from the seawater pool, and there was something about the water that I couldn't put my finger on. If I'd been in Copenhagen, I would have whipped out my phone to check if it was a bad day for water quality.

She gave a sad smile. 'The water in the fjord is not great, actually,' she said. 'It's affected by industry and farm run-off, overfishing, a large number of boats and there have been a lot of problems in recent years. The oxygen level is low, kelp is in decline and there is a specific type of mossy plant that blooms and suffocates all the plant life. Mussels, which used to thrive at the bottom of the fjord and act as cleaners, are disappearing. Waste is dumped into the harbour. The catalogue of things that shouldn't happen to a Scandinavian city are happening all over, and these layers of problems are leading to ecosystem collapse.'

I'm shocked. In fact, appalled. It's easy to take all these things for granted and sad to hear how bad things have got.

Siri and her friends have taken politicians out diving near the islands on the fjord, showing them in real time about how populations are declining. 'Some of them lived and grew up on the fjord, and are shocked to see how little life there is there today,' she said. They needed to see it for themselves before they took action. 'It definitely changed their heads and hearts. You have to see it with your own eyes and have it pointed out and discuss it to realise what's happening.'

Some projects are happening to stem this decline, but it feels so slow to me, coming from Copenhagen's harbour where water cleanliness is closely monitored, seals come to feast on the fish and urban farmers tend to strings of mussels in the heart of the city. A knowledge centre around urban plastic is being planned but it didn't feel like enough. Norway, country of big landscapes and dramatic vistas, seemed to have a bigger stake than most in keeping its water clean and its environment flourishing.

I told Siri about my theory that how you swim is how you do everything, and asked what she thought. She took a moment to consider it. 'Yes,' she said. 'I think that's right. My friends would say I swim gracefully and calmly. I know when I'm diving that I have to let go, get into flow and find peace to do it.'

I liked that approach – the idea that you can't push, you have to let it happen and find a flow. Siri's thoughtful response felt like part of the answer to the larger question I was asking all year: how do I navigate the world, and how can I do it better?

Going with the flow can be hard for me – I thrive on a little resistance. But going against it completely is exhausting and not sustainable. Finding flow could be the answer.

Siri thought a bit more about the idea. 'I love following my heart,' she said, 'following my intuition. You have to do that underwater, it's part of it. I also like to go deep into things when I'm at work, to lose myself down a rabbit hole – no,' she corrects herself, 'a whale road. That's how I am with things.'

I'm surprised a little that she talks about being a freediver in such a calm, considered way – it seems so risky, so adrenaline-filled and competitive to me. The idea of it being a place to go deeper into yourself, as well as going deeper into the water, is captivating. Perhaps all of us water-lovers are chasing something under the surface, something deeper than you might imagine at first glance.

17

Back home in Copenhagen, I tried my theory on Hanna's stepson, who was visiting and joined us swimming one morning. 'Is the way you swim the way you do everything?' I asked him. He thought for a moment. 'I don't like it when people put me under pressure to do things,' he said. 'I only want to do things when there's no pressure.'

It was the same with life as it was with swimming, he said – if he had to spend a day at the beach and the plan was to swim, he won't want to do it. He'd rather just come across it and do it than put that pressure around it.

It was interesting. I think I'm the opposite. I actively like the pressure. I ratchet it up and do things like this, deciding to swim once a week through a whole year, and diving from the deck into the water, rather than just thinking being in the water is enough, and climbing down the ladder and back up. I like swimming because the water washes away a lot of my stress, but my approach to swimming is to add more stress. I am the weirdest contradiction of all.

There are two ways to take this, for me. One is that I'm just returning to what I'm used to, to what I've been conditioned to in corporate life. These kinds of patterns, these modes of behaviours, get set in us, and even though they're bad for us, can feel comfortable and hard to break out of. The other way to see it is that I've recovered enough to be able to take on a bit more. On that first week of cold-water swimming, when I just went down the ladder and back again, I could never have done this. But I've rested and recovered. I'm braver and stronger. It's natural, then, that I'd start to push the boundaries and see how much more I can do. Like lifting weights at the gym, my courage has grown, my tolerance to the cold has improved and my lust for life is coming back. That's for sure. And maybe I'm just the kind of person who likes a bit of pressure too. But just the right amount, and not too much.

We were still swimming regularly, but one Wednesday morning, we convened on the wooden deck and looked at the water with a decided lack of enthusiasm. 'I was going to call you,' said Hanna. 'I don't really feel like swimming today. I'm just so tired.'

I knew how she felt. Having just taken one sad and tired child to school with leaden eyelids myself, all I wanted to do was crawl back into my warm bed. I knew in my heart that swimming would wake me up, but there was no point doing it if you didn't want to. We made a deal to check in with each other at lunchtime and maybe go then, if the looming dark grey cloud overhead had passed.

We were all really tired at that moment – teachers and kids, parents and colleagues. In a month's time it would be the equinox again, and the sun would be out in full force until 11pm. Even though it happens every year, the seasonal changes in Scandinavia have an impact on our bodies – a lack of dark/light cues make us stay up longer and try to stretch our energy later into the evening, and it's inevitable really that we would all be so tired. We all need to get better at this energy budgeting thing. There's a tide that moves against us when the days are darker, and a tide that pulls us along when the light comes back.

Something I've noticed with my kids is that they need nature and fresh air at least once a day. At the weekend, if they're still lounging about at home at lunchtime, they start, very slowly, to fray round the edges. Their energy turns inwards and they become snippy with each other. More often than not, it escalates into a full-blown fight in under an hour. I see it happening in me too. The thing that solves it is getting out into nature.

One Sunday, we take them to Refshaleoen, the post-industrial island in the north of Copenhagen where a former shipyard has been transformed into a leisure area. Where twenty years ago, you would have found hauliers and shipbuilders hammering in huge warehouses, sparks flying in smoke-choked air as metalworkers mended the huge ships that came in and out of the port, today there's a street food market that looks like someone has taken the food area from a festival field and put it on a wind-lashed concrete base next to a modern art gallery, several Michelin-starred restaurants, and a special little swimming spot called La Banchina.

La Banchina is painted a lovely turquoise colour, the shade you might choose for a tin of sardines or the hull of a sailboat, or, perhaps, the hand-glazed dinner plates in a seaside restaurant on a Greek island. It's the colour of a Hockney swimming pool, and that's a neat reference because of what it hides behind it. The tiny café-restaurant is off a busy, dusty road and backs on to the harbour, with decks and docks and a little garden with a round sauna and abundant greenery overlooking a still, deep pool of water, like a cul-de-sac from the main harbour. At the height of summer, boatloads of people turn up to this little harbour to drink and socialise; in the winter the lucky ones hunker down to six-course tasting menus inside. I haven't managed to get a booking there yet, but I live in hope. When we arrived, it was quiet, apart from three half-naked people running lightly across the grass, down to the deck, and into the water. You could almost hear the hiss of steam as they cooled off their sweating bodies in the water after the sauna. Then they were up and back into their warm pine-scented womb. One of the sauna rules here is that you are forbidden to scream when you jump into the water because the neighbours get annoyed; the sauna-goers were admirably restrained.

Sauna-less, I stripped off on the deck and climbed into the water, leaving my clothes in a puddle on the wooden deck. In the last few years, increased harbour traffic in Copenhagen has led to 'official' swimming zones being marked out with yellow buoys, to make it clear where you can and can't swim. A lot of them are monitored for water quality, giving an extra incentive to swim there, and all of them are off limits for watercraft. The swim zone at La Banchina is a small pocket of deep emerald green water, like a pond, underneath the sauna running from the deck to the wall, overhung with plants. It had a green flag next to it on my water quality app, meaning it was safe to swim.

A little seaweed clung to the metal ladder and the stone wall. It was not cold, not warm either, as I swam to the wall and back. The combination of the small restaurant, the garden and the deck makes this place feel special. You are not overlooked and you feel like you have a corner of the city all to yourself. It might not be so true when the overloaded yachts full of party boys steer into the little harbour in the summer, but it felt true as I trod water and swam back. I could almost have been in a river pool surrounded by weeping willows in an Oxfordshire river, it felt that secret. I got out and dove in a couple of times, unselfconsciously bobbing about in the clear water, feeling supported as it surrounded me. It was my only swim of the week so far, on a Thursday too, but it was worth the wait. I felt a great sense of well-being bubble up in me.

One day, while walking the dog, a realisation hit me. I'd been walking a narrow path lately, but I liked it. Travel, Write, Swim, Repeat pretty much covers it. Each of these ideas encompasses the things I love to do – travelling includes meeting new people and thinking about new ideas. Writing is of course writing, but it's also reading, researching, developing new ideas, collaborating. Swimming is swimming, but it's also doing things alone, and doing things with others. It's making new friends and it's finding a reason to talk to other people. I look at it from all angles. It is decidedly narrow. But it's making me happy right now, so I'm going with the flow. Crystallising things into this narrow funnel gives me some confidence, like I'm boiling myself down to my essence. It makes it clearer to decide what to do, now I know what makes me happy. And that's what I am. Happy, that is.

Things were working out in all sorts of ways that I hadn't anticipated. When I'd leapt out of my job, a net had appeared – the small, easy part-time writing jobs I'd been able to find in the city. But it hadn't taken long for my own freelance work to flourish and for me to feel that I could easily move on from them and make the life I wanted for myself. I was starting to feel that I could survive on my own. I put it down to the fact that the stories I was writing were the ones I wanted to tell – instead of stories that I thought my editors would want me to write. It's a subtle difference, but it's everything: having the confidence to share my view with the world instead of trying to fit theirs made it work. Boiling myself down to my essence, like I'd been doing all along, had a ripple effect. Being freelance is to walk a tightrope between too much work and not enough work all the time, with a fear underneath it all that you might fall into a chasm of penury and not be able to get out, but from somewhere, confidence was flowing that I'd get to the other side. I still wasn't quite sure what I'd find when I got there, or what I was walking towards.

I read an interesting quote about burnout, that it isn't about overworking, it's about investing emotionally in something and not getting a return on that investment.

It stayed with me.

I was investing in myself, at least, in finding out what made me happy and chasing that, and I was getting some returns. I was happy walking a narrow path that fitted in with my values, skills and interests. I was trying to find flow in it, like Siri, and see where it took me.

18

From the air, the rocky islands looked like smudges on my glasses, smuts on the window, scattered across the otherwise perfectly turquoise Gulf of Finland. They took clearer shape as we came in to land: some were forested, with small clearings, houses and tracks snaking through the lush greenery, others were nothing more than bare rock. I had a sense that I was entering the world of *The Summer Book*, the perfect jewel of a book that the Moomins writer Tove Jansson wrote 50 years previously about life on a tiny Finnish island. It was the reason I was going to Finland in the first place, to find out more about that world and its legacy. Seeing all these islands like disconnected little independent worlds beneath me made me feel like I'd stepped back in time.

A few hours and a short ferry ride later, I was sitting in a wooden cabin 50 metres from the sea thinking about swimming. More accurately, I was thinking about not swimming and if it was OK if I didn't swim at all. The sea was grey, flinty; the sky a pale blue cossetted with clouds. A diving bird popped up from the waves for a second before going down again, its beak glinting in the evening sun. Near it, a pale orangey-pink rock kept fooling me into thinking that there was someone swimming out there in the Baltic. It wa almost exactly the shape a large man would make if he were doing front crawl, raising his elbow up to a perfect triangle above the water as he breathed. There were lots of rocks in the water just outside my window, so many that I could see exactly how I could swim there. Earlier, the lady who owned the cabin had shown me where she sometimes swam, just a little further down the pine-scented track, off big slabs of flat rock. I couldn't see how deep it was there, or an easy access or return point. The wind was bracing. It was evening. I was not so sure I was going to swim in the Baltic Sea in Finland after all. On the horizon, near the isolated island where Tove Jansson had lived and worked, beacons flashed off and on all night.

The cabin I was staying in dated to the 1970s, just like Jansson's book, and had even hosted the writer many years ago. While it might have had literary history to boast about, it didn't have hot running water, though there was cold water in a sink out the front. The toilet was a composting one, just out the back, and the kitchen was compact, but because I didn't think things through as well as I might have done, I didn't have everything I need. I didn't have coffee, or milk, or butter. I did have crispbreads with a hint of aniseed from the local shop, plus an abundance of eggs and a loaf of what I thought was rye bread but was actually a kind of sweet tea bread. Dinner was a hopeless version of boiled eggs on cake, and so embarrassing that I was glad to be eating on my own. I had got lost earlier while trying to navigate Helsinki airport too, in another moment of failure that had me wondering who I thought I was, working as a travel writer in the first place. Then again, being lost can lead to some exciting paths forward and unexpected breakthroughs, in life as well as in travel writing, as I know all too well. I am full of silver linings, if not an internal compass.

I was in Finland to trace the steps of the Moomins writer for a story for a newspaper, but it was more than just a story to me. It was more of a personal quest, filled with moments of serendipity. I've loved the book for more than a decade, taking it out as each summer comes round to remind myself of the slow unfolding of life, the delight to be found in tiny details and the imaginative worlds inhabited by the aging, cynical grandmother and her shiny-eyed granddaughter, Sophia. I'd already trekked through the woods here and down to the shoreline, wondering if anyone had ever found a seal skull washed up by the tide like she did in the book. While I was wandering, I found a velour-clad bear toy, wet as though it had been washed by the tide when it last was high, and pocketed it, intending to ask the owner of the house if she'd lost it, and take it home to my children as a lost treasure if not. I thought coming to the archipelago where my favourite book was written might imbue me with a missing creative spark, or inspiration that I hadn't thought of. Instead, I just missed my family. It was so green it nearly hurt my eyes. Green grass, green trees, the neon green of the blueberry leaves low on the forest floor and the brightness of the new shoots at the end of the fir fronds. It was noisy too, with white-capped waves racing across the Gulf and red and white striped masts standing far out to sea.

I thought about swimming again the next day. I was scared, to put it plainly, in a way I hadn't been all year. I was scared of swimming here, scared for the first time not of the cold, because I knew I could deal with that, but of being whisked away by the water, of drowning out in the cold, unfriendly Gulf of Finland, where nobody would see me and nobody would know I'd drowned. Maybe I'd wash up lost and friendless on a lonely beach like the velour-clad bear. With a friend it would be different, but right now, the water looked deep and unfriendly. Maybe tomorrow. Since I didn't have a shower, it was my only option to get clean anyway. I was due in Helsinki at a sauna in two days' time, but I was not so sure where the sauna was and whether there would be a sea-swimming option there too. I wanted to swim in Finland to add another country to my list, and I didn't want to break my streak of swimming once a week, every week: the question was how.

I walked through the forest along another track in the afternoon, encountering a deer on the path that looked at me for a moment with its calm eyes before skipping gracefully into the brush. At the end of this track, Tove Jansson's niece Sophia, the inspiration for the six-year-old girl in the book, had a summer house and it was magnificent. The boat house alone was more than half the size of my flat; the other modernist wooden buildings that made up the complex were surrounded by manicured lawns and landscaped gardens, and there was a little greenhouse in the middle of them too.

I walked past it and down another path that led to a big boulder and a view of the sea. There was no path beyond the boulder so I jumped down from it and walked through the blueberry bushes. In a little clearing, I found a skull, picked clean. It was a young deer skull, missing its lower jaw. I kicked it over with my foot. It was a neat counterpoint to all the life I could see around me – the blueberry bushes weeks from coming into fruit, the song of the birds above me in the canopy, the roar of the sea. Everything was so vital here, but this reminded me to seize life while I could. I continued down towards the sea and discovered a wide half-moon shaped bay, with calm waters and a rocky and sandy beach. I stood and watched the waves gently wash over it.

Another walk took me to the original pilot's house. Earlier, my walking guide Lisbeth had explained that this was an important place in the islands until relatively recently – and that most ships passing this way would stop and pick up a pilot, a local man who knew the waters incredibly well, so they could avoid the rocky surprises that lie all along the coastline here in the Gulf of Finland. I couldn't imagine the responsibility those men must have felt, needing to be able to deftly navigate between the rocky islands and half-hidden skerries in all weathers on routes to Helsinki and St Petersburg. I'd done some research before my trip, looking back to 50 years ago, when Jansson's book was published. Over that period, the essential appeal of these islands seems not to have changed so much, at least to me, and I wondered about how the next 50 would treat them. As you might expect, the prognosis was not good. With sea levels set to rise, many of the rocky islands in the archipelago would become skerries, and many skerries would be sitting under water, ready to rip a hole in the bottom of any boat that came by. Fifty years is a long time – fifty years ago the Vietnam War was still ongoing, and a scientific calculator was considered a technological breakthrough – and I'd be an extremely old lady fifty years in the future.

Swimming had brought me here. The greater stillness in me, and greater appreciation of nature created by it, made me more aware of my surroundings. I felt more attuned and more able to enjoy and document the little things going on around me. I felt stiller in myself, with a calm that underpinned it all. My mind flashed back to the manic energy I'd had a year ago, the inability to concentrate on anything for more than a moment, let alone enjoy it. As I walked and took notes and thought about how I'd write the piece, I was sinking into the slower rhythms of Scandinavian life and recognising their values. I was feeling more in harmony with the early dawn and the long light evenings, and I felt like I had space and time to do what I needed to do. I wasn't rushed and I wasn't trying to run a race at someone else's pace. I had time to think.

In the evening, the lady who owned the cottage I was renting invited me for dinner with her and her husband. We talked a curious mixture of Swedish, Finnish, Danish and English together and somehow seemed to get along. She must have been 60, Anne-Maj, if not older, I thought. There was still a rim of dirt around her nails from her morning work – she runs a farm and sells the vegetables in the local markets as well as looking after five holiday cabins on the island of Pellinge. She started the meal with a shot of Myrsky, a word meaning 'stormy' in Finnish, a schnaps tasting a little of Jägermeister, slamming it back with all the gusto of a student.

It was a lovely evening, and after a dinner of new potatoes, locally caught and smoked salmon, and salad from her garden, we went to the sauna, a few steps away in the garden. Stoked up and with a tank of water above it, this sauna was the only place you could wash when staying at my cottage. The idea was that in the evening, you heat it up, sweat it out, swim in the sea if you want or otherwise wash off the sweat with the water that has heated in the stove-top tank.

We chatted in a polyglot of languages and I told Anne-Maj about my swimming habit. She took it as a statement of intent. So, we'll cool off in the sea, then, she said. I tried to back out of it – it was slippery, the sea was a little rough, maybe we shouldn't – but she had a determined look on her face. Wrapped in just a towel, wearing black flip flops (me) and red Crocs (her), we picked our way across the detritus of the high tide mark, through a marshy little area and out to the large flat rocks. She went in first, slipping down between the cleft of a rock where there was a triangular-shaped pool washed with water. She was in, and then out. I scrambled in too, and felt the release of the cold water. It was slightly tempered by the fact that I was actually naked in public again, and there was just no stylish way to get out of the water. We returned to the sauna, and repeated the whole affair, before rinsing off with the warmed water.

I sat, thoroughly warmed through and relaxed in the late evening, looking out of the window, and I saw an otter perched on a nearby rock, still as a statue. A blink of an eye later and it had slipped cat-like into the water, leaving barely a ripple. I wondered if I had imagined it.

I woke up the next day to the calmest millpond sea, views out to Klovharun, Tove Jansson's island, and a desire to swim and swim out in that blue channel, to swim to nearby islands and picnic on them, and to skim stones in the sea. It takes some time to decompress when you get out to the countryside, my Finnish friend Fredrik tells me later. It's a process, this gradual switching off of your busy mind and a sinking into the countryside rhythm. Sometimes it takes him the best part of a week, but that's OK because he might be out in the archipelago for three

IV. Summer

of the world to take three weeks' holiday in the summer, and to spend most of it in the country in a little cottage near the sea. It was an idyllic thought.

I remember a Danish colleague telling me that two weeks' holiday was not enough – she only really started to relax on week two, so always needed a third. My English upbringing makes me approach holidays in quite a different way: I want to be out experiencing big, exciting things, like sunny beaches, dramatic ruins and fast-paced cities, not cosy countryside cottages where there isn't much to do. I think of the time off as a chance to do something, not the chance to do nothing.

It made me think about what Leena in Finland had said about summer, how Finns look at those brief weeks of full-on summer as days you squeeze all the juice out of. The seasonality in Northern Europe determines how you live, how you approach each season, and what personality you bring out. In the summer, everyone is an extrovert.

I wondered if that had something to do with my energy levels. Even though it was sunny from 4am to past 9pm, and those days were lengthening even more as midsummer approached, I was tired. I was not really keeping up with the hard-living Danes, who seemed able to look after their children, go to work and socialise every night of the week. I was sinking into the sofa at 6pm. Maybe I did need to do nothing after all.

There was one silver lining in it all, though: I had recognised that my energy was low and I was doing or four weeks. It's just how summer is done here in Finland. I don't have that luxury this time, and on my last day in the Finnish archipelago and then its countryside, I drive slowly back to Helsinki, past pastoral scenes that look like oil paintings, little red houses perched on lakes, small wooden pontoons jutting out into water, and swans gliding by.

Once back in Helsinki, I visited Kulttuurisauna, a Finnish-Japanese sauna on the harbour, with a friend and contact, Leena. It was a beautiful spartan place, with showers and a large wood-fired sauna so hot it nearly steamed up my contact lenses, and a strong smoky smell that stuck in my lungs like tar. It was hot, so hot, in this little female-only room, but once again the thermometer was broken and I was left to guess. Maybe 90, I thought. Sweat was pouring down my forehead as Leena and I swapped swimming stories. I'd been in touch with her for work since earlier in the year, and was delighted that she had agreed to meet me to tell me more about sauna culture in Finland.

The saying goes that Norwegians are born with skis on their feet, and Finns are born in the sauna. It's literally true of the older generations in Finland, whose saunas were the cleanest rooms in the house, and metaphorically true of younger generations, who have a sauna at least once a week. Out at their simple summer houses for four or more weeks in the summer, there is often no bathroom, and taking a sauna, which heats the water you wash with as I've found, is the way you keep clean. It's not so much a spa treatment as it is a necessity. And I like that. In the city, you most likely have a communal sauna in your apartment block which you can book for an hour or so with your family whenever you like. At home in Copenhagen, we have communal kayaks and paddleboards, but I would give anything for a sauna too.

Finland is certainly part of Northern Europe, and has strong Scandinavian roots, with its two official languages being Finnish and Swedish, but it's not a Scandinavian country – that's just Denmark, Norway and Sweden. It was the happiest country in the world in the year I visited, a fact that seemed to baffle and bemuse every Finn I came across. They just don't see themselves that way, and don't have a focus on being happy at every opportunity. As far as I can work out, it's more about having a well-balanced and mixed society, a strong connection with nature, and a high degree of trust in public bodies, than it is about walking around with a big smile on your face all the time.

The idea about connection with nature was interesting to me. Seasons are markedly different in Finland than further south: I was visiting in summer, when the skies were a perfect blue and the days were endless. In summer, Leena told me, we don't sleep. I thought I knew what the winters must be like – short dark days and a lot of hibernation – but it was only when she told me what it was like bringing up her eldest child in the winter of 2010, pulling a Bugaboo through snowy streets in -25°C because he would only sleep in the pushchair, that I really realised how different life this far north was. I had a baby in the same year but I did not need snow tyres for my pushchair – I never even realised Bugaboo did them. It's not for nothing that the Finnish word *sisu*, meaning resilience, is how the national character is defined.

Numerous studies have proven the positive health effects of taking a sauna due to the soothing heat and relaxing steam, and also thanks to the social aspect. We sat chatting in the steamy, hazy room, alongside around ten other women of different ages, from child to sixty plus. According to an old Finnish proverb, 'If sauna, liquor and tar don't help, the disease is probably fatal.' These days, as they swerve away from drinking and smoking, Finns are left with the sauna.

Taking a sauna is not just about looking after your health; it's also about socialising with others. I've read that sauna evenings are common among friends, neighbours, students and work colleagues, which is of course a bit tricky for me as a nudity-averse Brit. Imagine spending evenings sweating nakedly in the sauna with your work colleagues! I have also heard that pivotal decisions in Finnish political and business life have often been made in the sauna, and think of all those sweating businessmen with nothing but a towel for their modesty. I suppose it's a place where you have to trust the people you are with – you and they quite literally show that you have nothing to hide while sitting on those slatted wooden benches. In the hotel where I was staying, there was a sauna for guests in the basement, and in the most beautiful suites, a private sauna for those lucky enough to be booking them. You can find a sauna even in the cheapest youth hostel in Helsinki – it's that central to culture in Finland.

After several ladles of water were poured on the sauna, and great waves of heat were released, breaking over us as we sat on the top level of the busy sauna, I was gasping to escape so we put on our swimsuits and headed outside. There, in a little courtyard with wooden seats and a little greenery, we climbed down a ladder and swam broad strokes out into Helsinki harbour. It was the colour of milky tea, and the view was of piles of sand and a construction site. It reminded me a bit of the industrial views I saw when swimming in the harbour in Oslo. As I was wondering whether the water was really clean enough to swim in, a seagull swooped down to the surface, plucked a small thrashing fish out, and soared off. That was my question answered.

I asked Leena why she started swimming in the harbour – she had been doing it through the winter too, including in swimming holes cut in the ice. It turned out it was the same reason as me – after the stress and difficulties during COVID, she just wanted to feel alive again. So far, so similar, though she was many times more hardcore than me. I'd never cut a hole in the ice to go swimming and I wasn't about to start a toughness competition with a Finn, but I noted that we were both of a similar age, and had a similar approach to life. The water brought us both back to life in a way, back to our selves. I ducked under, surprised at how unsalty the water was, and we went back into the sauna to sweat and chat some more.

Back in Copenhagen, clumps of seaweed were floating in the water outside my flat, but I took it as a good sign that there was life in there. There was no sign of jellyfish yet, after that first burst of tiny jellies all those weeks ago, but for sure they were coming. I took full advantage of the floating swimming pool and swam long, lazy laps of breaststroke in the middle of the week in an almost empty pool. From the deck I could see the checkerboard of the net slung beneath it, keeping out the bigger fish way down deeper than my feet could reach.

19

Summer had arrived in my little corner of Copenhagen. Instead of seeing people wrapped in warm scarves and knee-length puffer coats when I walked back over the bridge from my morning dip, there were more and more people walking around with a towel slung casually around their shoulders like me. Others paired a bikini top with shorts, or walked around in just a bathrobe with a swimsuit underneath. Everywhere I looked, people were swimming.

In the space of a week, I saw the red RIB of the boat patrol cruise our canals twice on the look-out for swimmers taking to the water in unapproved spots. It was like seeing a car park attendant come round the corner when you know your ticket is about to run out. The deck below our flat, usually full of picnickers, swimmers and suntanning bodies at this point in the year, was deserted as a result. But they would be back.

In a few weeks, the schools would be out for six weeks, and most office workers would be on holiday for at least half of them. It is not unusual in this part

something about it. It was a big change from saying yes to everything on the burnout rollercoaster I was riding before. I was seeking a bit more stillness and a bit more time to myself whenever I could grab it. I thought about feeding my creativity and my calm by doing less. It seemed to be making a difference, just a little one.

We convened in the mornings, Hanna, sometimes Kasia and an occasional other friend, and me at the floating swimming pool, where we tended to be the only visitors, well before the lifeguards turned up. We were there because it was easy, it was clean and the big orange jellyfish couldn't get through the nets that protect the pool. We also wouldn't get fined by the boat police if we swam there.

One Saturday, we swam and I asked: What do we do when we come swimming now? I mean, if our gasp reflex, the body's response to the cold shock, had gone – the temperature in the water now was 19°C and would climb to 21°C in the space of a week, warmer than the air – where was the challenge?

The others agreed that it was a bit less focused now that we were not fighting the cold, proving something to ourselves. We swam laps instead, and actually enjoyed the water, along with each other's company. My skin barely had goosebumps when we came out, and it started to look a tiny bit tanned, no longer pink. I practised diving from the deck and felt the water flow over me.

Things were going better all round, at work, at home, at play. It couldn't be underestimated how vast a change that was from how things had been. Some of it was surely down to the sun, and how it cast a positive glow on everything, including my mood.

Then, as always happens when life stars to go swimmingly, the gods threw a massive spanner in the works. In the space of three days, my husband and oldest daughter saw the doctor about serious health issues. The swiftness of the respective doctors' actions took my breath away, speaking, as it did, of the seriousness of it all.

I tried really hard to carry on and support them, being as patient and as thoughtful as I could, but it was not long before I started to feeling bone-tired, tearful, fearful and desperate about it all. I was panicking about how to look after my most loved people in the world, and feeling deep inside myself that I wasn't up to scratch, that I couldn't do it, that I might let them down. I couldn't swim away these feelings; the only thing I thought was that I could cry underwater and nobody would know.

I cried when I took the dog for a late evening walk in the gathering dusk, hoping I wouldn't bump into anyone I knew. I didn't want anyone else in my house to feel like I couldn't cope or that they had caused my inability to cope – they needed someone strong and reliable so they had space to recover. I took a deep breath and put one foot in front of the other and did my best, even though it felt like it almost certainly wasn't good enough. Before the end of term,

I had a birthday party to host, a school sleepover to attend, and an away day with work, plus a bunch of school meetings and more doctor appointments. It was two weeks to get through. I would have to give the bare minimum to each of these activities just to get through it, as most of my energy was going into worrying, but I would do it. I had to.

I skipped a couple of swim sessions with Hanna, but also reflected that she knew what it was like, having endured a deeply sad few months recently too. She had found that swimming helped – and I know it's good for me too, but my mind felt too busy to give into it as much as I'd have liked. On windy days, the water looked as harried as my mind and I felt the bravery needed to jump in elude me. I needed a calm, sunny day and an empty hour to reconnect with the water, but they were hard to find. One sunny Wednesday morning, I walked round the harbour to the floating swimming pool to meet Hanna. She was looking into the water closely, peering into its clear depths, where great blades of seagrass rippled in the current.

'Jellyfish,' she said. 'There are jellyfish everywhere.'

She was right. A translucent jellyfish outlined in white, the size of a dinner plate, floated by as I watched. In the swimming area itself, the pool was dotted with pale orange jellyfish, trailing their long tentacles behind them. The tentacles were pale, white and somehow stomach-curdling, a sight that made me think of tendrils of egg white escaping a boiling egg and flowering into water. The umbrella-shaped bells would have been pretty, frothy like a many-petalled rose or a tulle skirt, if they had been attached to a more benign creature.

I had never been stung by a jellyfish. Some people say it's like being stung by a nettle. I didn't think these ones were big enough to worry about, but all the same, a couple of older ladies were taking their morning swim in the seaweed-clogged junior pool, where the water only came up to your waist and a perforated plastic bottom kept most of the wildlife out. There weren't any lifeguards around to ask whether it was dangerous or not, or to help us if it was. There hadn't been any warnings around the harbour or on local news either, so maybe it was fine.

I climbed down the ladder, surprised at the cold, and swam as quickly as I could to the other side. Hanna stood on the deck on jellyfish watch and warned me when I came too close to a pastel orange specimen the size of a tangerine. Its limbs trailed more than three times its body size behind it. Then I was out. Job done. Except it didn't feel like it. It was not fun, and it was not satisfying, and it kind of sucked. Hanna wouldn't swim with me; she's petrified of them. We had been swimming since the bitter winter and now that the glorious summer opened out ahead of us, the jellyfish were getting in the way.

Later, I looked them up and learned that there are only two types of stinging jellyfish in these waters: the lion's mane, an orange-red jellyfish with trailing tentacles, which I'd seen, and the blue fire jellyfish. Regardless of their colour, stinging jellyfish are called '*brandmænd*' – firemen – in Danish. There is also a translucent-white jellyfish which is called a 'water men', or '*vandmand*', but it is harmless. Of the stinging jellyfish, I read that they are unpleasant to touch and can ruin a day at the beach, but aren't considered truly dangerous, just like a stronger, longer-lasting nettle sting. They are most common in the late summer. If you do get stung, the advice is to scrape off any trace of jellyfish, douse the area with vinegar and then soak in hot water.

Halfway through my year of Scandinavian swimming, the last thing I wanted to do was to stop now. I opted to add a few extra vinegar bottles to my cupboard and just keep swimming.

While I was battling family health matters along with the jellyfish, hope arrived in the shape of my old business coach, who emailed me for a chat. He had been off the radar for a while, but not because he had been busy, as I'd suspected, but because he was burned out. He writes a blog about mindfulness, business advice and interesting businesspeople, and a post popped up on it all about his situation. In it, he wrote: 'My burnout was not from physical tiredness. It's caring and investing and hoping for things and not getting that. Over and over again.'

We talked a little about it all, comparing notes on this feeling of sadness, disappointment and exhaustion. Like me, he had self-diagnosed his burnout. He asked how it affected me and why I thought it was something more than tiredness and stress. I had to think about it. It seemed to have taken place in another lifetime. I replied that I thought it was in the impaired decision making more than anything else. It had been hard to have a clear thought, to make good decisions. I had stomach ache all the time, but that might have been because I was so busy that I couldn't eat properly, which then had all these physical effects. My brain was whirring on a constant motor and at no point did I feel able to stop and review what I was doing. I was just on, on, on.

I think as well as caring and investing and not reaping rewards for what I was doing, the whole machinery that was driving me onwards instead of reviewing and calibrating was causing the problem. I was not a machine, I was a person, and I needed to build in points to review, consider and think along the way too. I never stopped to celebrate something done well, or fix something that had gone wrong. It was just forward, onward, all the time.

I told him that I felt now that some of the fault lay with me. I wished I'd had a manager who could have spotted it and supported me too, but from what I could see, all the more senior people to me had their own problems to deal with anyway. My thinking had shifted on this for sure. My lack of boundaries made me a sitting duck for burnout, and I didn't sit and think about what I needed to do my job well. I was moving forward without any of this thinking and planning, and I didn't feel I could say no, but I could have and should have, repeatedly.

He nodded, in recognition. I felt sad for him and for myself, and for anyone going through it: this whole rollercoaster, this warp-speed ride that work had been for me until recently, with a focus on productivity over quality, is completely bent out of shape. One good thing: it was not how I saw things anymore.

Finding a way to find value in my own work, beyond worrying about whether it has been successful or not, has been a key element in pulling me out of it, I know that. So too has spending time thinking about what sets me alight and what doesn't. There's something to be said for being surrounded by the right people as well, a support network or friends or a scene that you fit into. All of these things help.

On the same day, I got an email from Karin the mermaid about swimming together again, and I was in a reflective mood. What a joy to have started on this swimming project. What a joy to be surrounded by people who like to swim. I wanted to say yes to all of that.

The next Monday morning I hit a new swimming area in Teglholm with Hanna, a short walk around the quay on my island. This little complex of pools was brand new, freshly opened this summer, and included a little square concrete-bottomed pool with mesh sides for smaller children, a slightly deeper version of the same, and then a roped-off area beyond it with a row of yellow buoys dividing the swimming lane from the main harbour area, where the speedboats and paddleboarders range. We walked along the deck looking closely for jellyfish before we disrobed, but there was nothing there. We were the only people disturbing the inky water. I stood on the diving board for a few minutes, looking down at the navy-blue water. The sky was dark grey, the temperature was around 12°C, and there was a light wind.

Normally I wouldn't hesitate, but there was something stopping me. The diving board was all wrong. Unless I dove in really shallowly and pulled up quickly, I'd end up surfacing under the yellow buoys on the wrong side of the line. It didn't really matter – it was not as though there were many speedboats around at 8am on a Monday morning – but it annoyed me. You see, that's what happens when you spot a single example of imperfect design in Denmark. Everything is so good here 99 per cent of the time that one misstep made me react in the most ridiculous way. I went down the ladder instead and swam a couple of laps round, feeling irked to begin with, until the feeling washed away. After the second dip, everything washed away and I was ready to start the week with my best foot forward.

I saw my doctor for a quick catch up about my daughter's situation and how I was dealing with two family health crises at once. She was, as always, amazing: thoughtful, kind, empathetic and ready to share some great ideas. Her best stress-fighting idea was strangely familiar to me. She played me a YouTube video of a Buddhist monk talking about the monkey mind and how to slow it down with a breathwork meditation. It is a classic stress-fighting technique – in essence, when you start feeling overwhelmed, you bring all your focus to your breath, so your concentration can't scatter into a thousand pieces and make you feel out of control. You breathe in, count to four, then breathe out, in a box-breathing fashion. Four counts in, hold it for four counts, four counts out, hold it for four counts. It has a remarkable way of clearing your mind, recentring your attention and stopping those spiralling thoughts.

Why did this feel so familiar?

That's right, it was because gaining breath control was what my friend Christina advised me to do on my very first winter swim. I practised staying in the water until I was in control of my breathing and it felt incredible. Being in such cold water brought everything back to one thing: breathing. It's like wiping the slate completely clean.

The other thing the doctor suggested was to take a slow walk and revel in my senses. Hear the crunch of gravel under my Birkenstocks. Look at the patterns of light the leaves leave on the ground, and feel the breeze on my skin. It was another way to calm down and realign yourself, putting yourself in a new context that is not wholly in your messy, stressy and confused head.

Leaning into the senses was familiar too – it was forest bathing, but in the city. And I was glad for the reminder to practise it more.

I tried the breathing when I was feeling stressed or pulled in too many directions, and it helped every time. When I had a house full of noisy twelve-year-old girls at the end of June, when I had a weekend packed with friends to see and shopping to do, and when I spotted a client I'd like to work for and sent them an introduction email, I stopped and breathed and cleared my head, and things didn't seem so insurmountable after all.

One Saturday afternoon, on my way home from a friend's house, I sank into the sensory approach. I was cycling past the back of a cemetery, and the greenery was escaping its bounds, long arms of brambles reaching out as if to grab me and pull me in, and fronds of trees and other plants leaning into the bike path like a crowd beside a race stretching out for a high five. There was a blackbird somewhere, singing loudly from the treetops. Suddenly life felt a bit easier to handle. Despite everything, there were moments of sunshine to enjoy.

I looked out of the window on a 30°C Sunday morning, the water glittering in the sunshine and speedboats cruising to and fro. It was a heavenly spot. I made a snap decision: I was going to swim across the harbour, from one side to the other. It was not legal – the lifeguards in the red boat would definitely fine me if they saw me – and I needed to find the right spot, so I would not put myself in the path of the yellow harbour bus or the many other boats zipping all over the place. But I was going to do it and I was going to enjoy it, jellyfish or no jellyfish.

There was a low bridge that crossed the harbour, so low that the harbour bus couldn't sail under it, and it had to be opened to let the occasional taller ship through. I spied a point on the deck from where I could slip down a ladder into the water and swim to the other side, where houseboats made from reconditioned ferries and fishing boats parked in a long line. These houseboats were gorgeous, with great sunny decks and enormous living rooms inside, stretching the length of the boat, with sleeping quarters underneath. Next to one of the houseboats, there was a workshop that I'd had my eye on for a while. Constructed from a floating wooden platform and with wonky-looking windows all along it, the owner used it as a woodworking studio, but I'd love to use it as a writing studio, so I could stare out on to the harbour from a metre above it whenever I was searching for a phrase or trying to find just the right word from the depths of my mind. It was a dream and it most likely would stay one, but I liked the idea.

I dragged my husband, dog and kids along to watch me swim – because even though there were other people in the water, I was swimming on my own across this 100 metre stretch and I didn't have a bright swim hat on or a colourful float bobbing in my wake, and boats could come at you from anywhere, appearing from the little canals and the marinas along it at any time. There was also the jellyfish thing. Even though I hadn't seen a big orange jellyfish in the harbour yet, only ones the size of a tangerine, it didn't mean they weren't there.

The seaweed was waving around the ladder as I climbed down into the water. I switched on my underwater camera, keen to see what else was in the water as I swam, and pushed off. There was a light current, not much of a breeze, and the water was around 19°C. I looked back briefly and saw my husband in conversation with one of our friends, who was also on the platform. I'd be looking out for boats on my own, then.

I swam a swift breaststroke through floating wreaths of seaweed and patches of cold water, then patches of warm water. At every stroke, my fingertips were alive to the thought of jellyfish and my feet were aware of the great cold depths beneath them where the big fish live. I focused my eyes on the bright orange ladder on the other side. A hundred metres is nothing, but it was my first island-to-island swim. And hopefully not my last.

I reached the ladder and paused for a moment. There were drifts of seaweed all around it, but not much else. I was keen to get back across without being stopped by the boat police and was already mentally preparing a pathetic and untrue 'sorry, I didn't know, I'm English' apology speech if I was caught. I swam back again a little more relaxed, waiting for a white pleasure boat to pass by as I did. The occupants were reclining on brown leather seats drinking wine, and barely gave me a glance as they powered by. I picked up the pace through the blue-green water and then I was there, back at the original ladder, climbing out.

A year earlier, I'd never have done this. I was a little bit delighted that I could still find new things to do in the harbour.

20

More swim-travel plans were in the air in July as I started to pull together a nearly two-week trip of a lifetime to Greenland that would also take in Iceland, bringing together work, a conference and some top-of-the-world swimming. But before I could get myself fully prepared or in the mood, the summer holidays were upon us.

While my husband was working, I took the kids on a mini adventure one Friday afternoon, packing our bikes with our lightest tent and three sleeping bags, forgetting half the tent pegs, to a campsite on the other side of the city. We cycled there, stopping for ice cream on the way at Svanemøllen beach, where I swam with Karin the mermaid all those months ago, then continued on to Charlottenlund beach, where the campsite was hidden inside an old fort looking out to sea. Charlottenlund Fort was built in the late 1800s to protect Denmark from the sea and fortify Copenhagen against invasion. It has been disused for over a hundred years, but when we turned up, there were invaders aplenty.

The sea was blue and the waves were calm. There was a shimmer of Sweden on the horizon, and in between the two bodies of land, white sailboats skimmed across the perfectly flat blue sea. As we got closer, we saw why, despite the perfect conditions, the water was curiously empty of people. There was not a single child dipping their toe in the water, and not a single adult swimming out in the great blue. A million tiny things were stopping them.

The tideline was blistered with little jellyfish, with pale orange beads of colour woven into the dark seaweed at the edge of the water, and bloated white blobs washed further up the beach, stranded by the tide. My swimsuit stayed balled in a towel in my bag.

I was disappointed. I'd spent the previous five days out of the water with an ear infection, looking forward to this day. But it wasn't to be. We ate pizza on the grass beside the beach, and played catch until the sun started to pale in the sky, before retiring to our tiny tent to sleep.

The next day, on the bike ride home from our one-night adventure, I broke the no-swimming spell back at Svanemøllen beach. The weather was perfect. The sand was clean and jellyfish free. A yellow buoy, maybe 75 metres offshore, bobbed about invitingly. As the lifeguard station had a blackboard saying that there were strong winds but nothing else to worry about, I got into my swimming costume, left the kids playing catch on the beach and stepped into the water.

At Svanemøllen, you have to wade a long way out to be able to start swimming. My eyes raked the sand under my feet, looking for anything that could be a jellyfish. But there was nothing. Soon enough, the water hit my waist and I was swimming, heading out to the nearest buoy, with green water beneath me and sand beneath it. There was a drop-off where I rounded the pier and the water went from green to black, and it got colder. Tendrils of seaweed grasped at my feet, my ankles, my wrists. I knew it was nothing but seaweed, but I felt a cold stab of fear inside me. My new swimming costume had adjustable ruching so I could make the legs as high or low as I liked, and it trailed the cords that adjusted the sides down my legs. My body was already hyper-alert to the possibility of the trailing tentacles of a large jellyfish and that was not helping. Then the wind picked up, blowing spray into my face.

I started to think about the bottom of the sea reaching up, trying to claim me and pull me down, wrapping me in its long grass-like tentacles until I couldn't break free. Dark memories of the Viking exhibition and the goddess with the seaweed-like hair didn't help. I was three quarters of the way out to the buoy but I bailed. I swam back to shore as quickly as I could, as if chased by something from the depths. Ran wasn't going to keep me today. It wasn't the greatest way to break my no-swimming spell, but at least I was back in the water. It got me over my bigger unvoiced worry: what if I got used to not swimming and never went back, breaking my promise to myself to swim once a week every week through the year?

I'd already got so far but I didn't completely trust myself to keep on doing it. Every time I stood on the deck looking at the water, or on a beach, or at a swimming platform, there was a tiny voice in my head saying, *But what if you* don't *do it?* I had succeeded in drowning her out for a long time, but she was always there. Some days she was louder than others. Some days I felt stronger than others. As I got further away from corporate life, and found myself more in this new life, my motivation to keep going waned, maybe because the need to keep doing it felt less urgent. Underneath it all, I was still a bit a bit scared, not of the water, but of failing myself, and not sticking to the plan. I didn't want to feel like it had all been for nothing.

I met Mags at a work party in Sweden and immediately knew she was going to be fun. Within a few hours of meeting each other we'd shared a love of swimming and hatched a new plan. She invited me to her island in the Stockholm archipelago with a great idea: we should swim round it. 'It takes about two and a half hours,' she said, 'and there are no jellyfish. How about coming over in August?'

Over the next two weeks, it became all I could think about. Even though I had a 'swimming in Greenland' project bubbling away in my mind, the idea of swimming round a Stockholm island seemed more exciting. The idea of a longer swimming challenge fired me up, even as the rest of my brain was sitting on a deckchair relaxing. I told a few friends and their faces told me that planning to swim for over two hours in one go was not a normal thing to be thrilled about.

'Do you really think you can swim that long?' asked one.

I shrugged. 'Of course,' I said. 'I mean, I think I can. Probably not very quickly. But I'm sure I can. I can, right?'

Her face disagreed. Doubt starts to creep in. Perhaps I was getting ahead of myself.

There was only one way to tackle this uncertainty: I decided to prove to myself that I could. I liked swimming. I didn't really love swimming in a chlorinated swimming pool, but the hypnotic, meditative state I could get into when swimming lengths could be enjoyable. I thought about cycling to the pool one summer evening to swim for an hour, to prove to myself that at the least I could do that, but when I checked the schedules, I found that the indoor swimming pools were closed for summer. Swimming pool attendants needed a three-week holiday too, it seemed.

I settled myself to swim in the floating pool in the harbour, with its asymmetric basin that I could sort of squint at and pretend it was like swimming lengths. It was about 25 metres across, 19°C in the water and in the air, and there were no obvious jellyfish. I put on my long-sleeved swimsuit, with the thought that it might keep me a tiny bit warmer, and I climbed down the ladder gingerly, still suffering from an ear infection, to swim 50 lengths. My eldest daughter, who didn't want to swim too, set my stopwatch on the deck and went home as I started a ladylike, leisurely breaststroke. I was not in a rush: this wasn't a race, it was an endurance test, after all. I just wanted to know if I could swim for this long, for this far, just to start with.

Ten lengths in and my hands had started to cramp a little. It had been a while since I'd swum properly like this. Even though I swam all the time, I didn't do lengths or great distances very often. It was usually more about being in the water than powering through it. I rested my hands for a few seconds and then tried again.

Thirty lengths in and a light chill was starting to set in. I swam up and down, up and down, past kids jumping in off the side, sending ripples across the surface of the water. The wind blew horizontally, so swimming in one direction was easy and the other was a more of a fight where water sprayed into my face and little waves rose up and washed my top lip. I did a smooth breaststroke, the sort you would swim if you had done your hair and make-up and didn't want to mess it up. I had not done my hair and make-up, and even if I had, I would rather have fun than worry about messing it up, but I didn't want to get any more water in my sore ear than necessary. Anyway, I was never one for that kind of dynamic, flashy and undulating style of breaststroke, where you bob up and down in the water like a duck. It was calm Sunday swimming, the equivalent of Sunday driving, all the way for me.

Around the edges of the pool, people were sitting, sunbathing, gossiping, scrolling their phones and hanging out. It operated as a de facto park for our area, and not everyone came to swim. Just because the local park has a football pitch, it doesn't mean you have to kick a ball around. Just because there was a pool in the middle of our park, it didn't mean everyone wanted to swim. There was nobody that I knew or recognised there that day, though.

The harbour bus kept coming and going into the harbour channels, all the time I was swimming, rocking the floating wooden structure and sending bulges of water rippling across the pool. An older lady with a beautiful dark blue octopus tattoo on her forearm jumped in like a teenager with a splash. A man, her husband perhaps, adjusted his swimming goggles and swam a few splashy lengths of front crawl before climbing out and reading a book on the deck.

Three twentysomethings arrived, got changed and then hesitated on the side. The man went to get a net and the girls pointed into the deep green water at the other side of the pool from where I was swimming. He scooped something out – an orange jellyfish, I guessed – and then they all climbed down the ladder, squealing at the cold, for a brief dip.

All the while, I kept swimming up and down, up and down. I stopped, panting briefly, after each set of ten, and then set off for ten more, wishing I had a firm side to push against instead of the nylon net that hung under the deck to keep the big fish out. I was not tired and my hand wasn't cramping any more, but I was growing cold. The outer layers of my body were getting really cold, but I was still moving and panting and pushing forwards. It was as if my cold skin belonged to someone else. I was disassociating from my body as I swam, which was probably a bad sign.

I reached 50 lengths and thought about continuing. I was not tired; I was rolling at a pace I could keep up for a lot longer. But I was curious about how long it had been, and I was definitely getting colder.

My fingers fumbled the stopwatch, which said 45:01 Not even an hour. The sun was shining warmly on the deck but the wind was cold, so I changed smartly out of my swimsuit and into my clothes and walked around the harbour back home. I wrapped myself up in a blanket and found some woolly winter socks to heat my feet back up to the usual temperature as I sat on the balcony later.

One thing was glaringly obvious to me after my first trial of longer distance swimming: I was going to have to get a wetsuit. For a longer swim, it was just a fact. It didn't mean I'd use it when I was swimming the rest of the time. I wouldn't. I didn't like being squeezed into a neoprene tube; it meant that you felt the water differently. You were separated from it via this black fabric barrier. I'd rather swim naked all the time than swim in a wetsuit. The feeling of the water on your skin, the sense of being able to stretch all your limbs, that notion of being part of the water and part of nature was lost as soon as you insulated your body in a wetsuit. But I thought for this one challenge, it was going to be difficult without one.

There was another thing too: I was right not to be daunted by a two-and-a-half-hour swim. I still needed to train for it, and planned to do a number of other swimming sessions like this before I headed to Stockholm. But it was a really enjoyable 45 minutes, and with the energy of added company like Mags, I was confident I could do it three times over.

21

Before Greenland, which was now booked in and definitely happening, I still had another place to visit. In July, I packed the craziest suitcase I'd ever packed for a family summer holiday. In it went two fishing nets, two crab fishing poles, a small life jacket, two wetsuits, four packets of cake mix and some seriously thick jumpers. We were off to the Arctic Circle, where the whales roam and sea otters play, and there were no cars and no shops. I couldn't wait. The rest of Europe was in meltdown mode, with record temperatures and liquifying roads; in Fleinvær, the only roads are liquid ones anyway, and the only cars are boats. We were going to the Arctic Hideaway together, the scene of my frog skin sauna meltdown and my snowy trip earlier in the year. After the health scares and stress of the last few weeks, perfect calm on an island miles from anywhere was just what we needed to recover.

Four months on, there was still snow on the distant mountain tops. I wondered if it had fallen when I was last there, in that freezing cold March that felt like years ago. Where there were snowdrifts, there were now verges and valleys filled with wildflowers and long grass and drifts of white flowers, angelica, up the side of the highest hill. Håvard greeted us as old friends, and over the next few days, we fell into a routine with his friend and their children, of eating, cooking and living life at a slower pace. There was no need to rush, after all – the daylight went on and on. It was July and on a clear day, the sun barely set, colouring the sky with a haze of pink and orange instead as it dipped behind an island and came back up again rather than setting and reappearing like it does in the rest of the world. One night it made a deep pink slash in the sky like a wound.

The unreal daylight and lack of night lulled us into a dreamlike rhythm. We got up at ten and went to bed after midnight. We ate when we were hungry, and slept when we wanted. We alternated fishing, sitting in the sauna, swimming in the chilly water, and combing the shoreline for orange and purple sea urchin shells. The water was still bone-chillingly cold, even on a sunny day. On days when the wind blew from the north, it felt like the breath from a frozen giant. It all felt like a dream, like stepping into an alternate universe where the balance was changed.

The salt water was refreshing. I dove into the Arctic Sea headfirst, reaching out beyond the deck to where the kelp blew in the current beside the occasional orange jellyfish. Then I swam straight back, feeling the cold steal into my toes. It was painful – I couldn't stay in any longer if I'd wanted to. It was just as cold the second or third time. The kids climbed down the ladder to dip and then raced off again. My sensible, reliable, unfailingly kind husband was goaded into jumping off the sauna pier, down three metres into the ocean, by a Norwegian boy with long hair and a cheeky manner. Then he did it again. It was an unexpected burst of impetuousness from him: the Arctic brings out an adventurous side in everyone. In the deeper water, we saw dark purple skinny-legged sea stars lying on the rocks and the sand, and great round globes of spiny sea urchins perched on the kelp.

I had the sense, the whole time we were there, that we were going through a rewilding. Alone one morning, I climbed the highest hill on my own past hip-high cow parsley, little patches of bright yellow cowslips and red clover up to my shins. At the top, I sat on the bench and scanned the sea with binoculars, seeking life in and under the water. Geese honked in the background, Arctic tern wavered by on the breeze, and I focused out beyond the last island to the deep blue beyond where the whales lived. There was nothing but navy waves and white horses to see as far as the horizon, but I dreamt a little about what life lay beneath.

My eye took in the contours of a tiny island at the back of the hill, with little white flowers growing at the top, bright white patches of guano and a kelp skirt. On the top, fixed into the rocks, there was a rusted hoop where a boat could be tied up. In the far corner, a little beach and a tiny brown rock at the back that seemed to be moving. But it was not a rock. It was the oiled contours of an otter, eating something small. I watched it for a few seconds, noting how closely it blended with the brown rocks around it, unsure if it really was an otter and not a rock. Then it calmly stood up and slipped into the water.

It was my fourth otter sighting of the year. Every one seemed just as magical, just as unbelievable. A glimpse of this shy creature felt like a reward for slowing down.

There was a real magic to the days we spent on this little 1.4 kilometre-long island. I walked the full length of it with my smallest daughter one day, past an odd grey municipal lamppost, as out of place as the lamppost beyond the wardrobe in Narnia. With no night right now, there was no need for artificial light. Well, not for a month or so, anyway. The clouds lay heavy on the horizon, making the sea hard as flint, unswimmable, so we contented ourselves with a nature walk instead. We walked in sandals along the grassy path and down to the first bridge where slippery rocks led to a beach strewn with shells. The tide was out and crab claws lay like the discarded bones from a feast along the shoreline. Tide pools were fringed with a feather-boa-like neon-green seaweed.

We searched for treasures, picking our way along the white sand and into the cold, clear water. Green-backed crabs crouched under rusted pieces of metal;

sun-bleached seaweed looked like the remains of a party-popper streamer. A sandpiper stood long-legged on a telephone wire calling out a warning to anyone who would listen. We found periwinkles, shiny top shells, small scallop shells and the smashed remains of an orange sea urchin. Pairs of clam shells and cockles caught my daughter's eye, along with rock quartz that she pocketed for her sister, who loved a mystical crystal.

On the way back, we walked past a house with a bumpy but manicured lawn mowed by a pair of robot lawnmowers. It was strangely unnatural in this landscape of mountains and wildflowers to see the wildlife controlled so intensely and intensively. And the robots were definitely out of place. Delicate harebells waved in the breeze and stubborn little yellow flowers clung to rocks but not in this garden, which was green and grassy and almost as neat as a cricket pitch, if it weren't for the contours. It was more like Astroturf than natural grass. In this wild and beautiful place, I found it baffling, an affront, even. I wanted to throw the damn things into the sea.

The ghost of the conversations I had in the sauna with Jarl and Laura in March drifted back to me when I fired up the wooden cave of a sauna later. Four months on, life felt more than a little different. I was still trying to find my balance, but I was more sure-footed than before. I was a stubborn little flower clinging to the rocks, and a bit less like a shallow-rooted flower spinning out in drifts across a hillside. An extra four months of swimming had brought me more focus and determination, and a greater appreciation for nature. Some days I felt like I was flourishing, even, something I couldn't have imagined back in the days when I was schlepping to work and suffering under artificial lights; on others I still felt as if I was sinking like one of the crabs that fell off the ferry quay earlier, down to the unknown depths. More often than not, though, I was just floating through it all. And these days, unlike this time last year, I had time to drink, eat, think, plan. Burnout was starting to feel like a memory, especially in this place. My senses felt rinsed clean like a city street after rain. I would never have dived headfirst into the sea last time I was here; now I was doing it multiple times a day. How time, and nature, heals all.

The kids found a home at the studio of Are Andreassen, a Norwegian-Sami artist specialising in graphic prints and lino cuts. A tall man with a wide and gentle face under a broad-brimmed black hat, a thin white ponytail snaking out from the back, he was the grandfather of the boisterous boys who had been hurling themselves into the water from the sauna dock. He possessed oceans of patience. His mustard-yellow studio looked out to the sea along a path from the Arctic Hideaway. Above it, two flags flew: the Norwegian flag and the Sami flag. Are's mother was Sami and he told of how his family members had been banned from speaking their language in the past and forced to assimilate into Norwegian culture, leaving huge tranches of their traditions and culture behind. These days, Sami paintings hang on the walls of the new national gallery in Oslo and represent Norway at the Venice Biennale, but the spotlight is relatively new.

Are's studio was a treasure trove hung with black and white prints, curios like a huge, dried King Cod, and artworks by his talented family and visitors. Within hours, the children were hooked on lino cutting, drawing and then carving out swirling pictures of sea otters and waving seaweed on the grey surfaces. Cutting lino isn't just about technical skill and composition; it's about creating an image that will work in two colours, black and white, there and not there. Prints are strong and bold, stories told with light and dark. It's a story of all the people living in this part of the world, where the light and dark are balanced and unbalanced through the year, and extremities are easily felt. There is no grey area – it either works or it doesn't. Creating these works is both simple and complicated at the same time, conceptual and graphic, detailed and bold.

We saw more of Are's work in the evening, in a packed island clubhouse where his ex-wife, an exceptional folk musician, was performing. She stamped the floor passionately with her feet as she played the fiddle, then captured the audience as she told stories of wedding marches led by a violinist around the islands, and birds and their distinctive calls. Above her, as she played and sang music that reminded me of a lark in flight over a meadow of wildflowers, floated a black and white flag, primal and dark like life lived here, on the edge. It depicted the ancient tribal shape of a sea monster with twisted arms and clawed legs and the teeth of a terrible pike.

I asked Are about the sea monster banner the next day, and he told me he came up with it one day with his grandson when they were talking about a development in Norwegian fishing.

'You know they are going to start fishing for those small creatures – what are they called, the ones that feed all the fish?' he said, groping for the English words.

'Krill?' I said.

'Yes, krill,' he said. 'It's a test project but they are investing heavily in it so you know what that means. They will be fishing for krill and using them to feed the fish farms. Nobody is talking about it. There may be unintended consequences – we don't know what else is out there. And we were talking about that, and came up with this idea of a sea monster.'

The big wooden printing plate he used for the giant monster was leaning against the wall, taller than my daughter. The conversation wandered and we didn't return to it, so I was left thinking to myself: Was this clawed sea beast an ancient creature woken by the krill fishermen, with its sharpened nails ready to attack and protect its deep and formerly impenetrable home? Or were the real monsters the nakedly grasping people who were allowing it all to happen, putting profit before nature? Environmental protection in the wildest, most vulnerable places in the world like northern Norway seemed to be lacking, right when it was needed the most. Perhaps it was because there were not enough people there to speak out, and nature can't speak for itself.

I looked out of the window and thought about the killer whales, the black and white orca, seen in the fjord earlier in the year, and the hulking hull of a cruise ship I saw days before, larger than an island, more populated even in its kitchen than the whole 300-island archipelago we occupied. Some issues were plainly black and white.

We spent our last few days in much the same way, day merging to dusk, night never arriving, the pace of life as slow as a snail. I thought how in overheated Copenhagen, the week before we travelled, slipping into the empty harbour bath at the end of the day was blissful, like slipping into cool silk sheets. Here, not so much. Only after layering the sauna oven with cardboard and egg boxes, shavings of wood and small logs, leaving it for an hour or two, and sitting in it for ten minutes, was I was able to contemplate the Arctic waters, and then only for a few moments. The smoke signal of the sauna called Are's grandsons to join us and they whooped along the quay, lifejackets on, to jump into the cold water with gusto, but I was still tentative, slipping in via the wooden ladder rather than jumping in straight from the top.

Back in the kitchen, wildflowers dropped their petals on the table, curling up at the edges. We sat in the late afternoon sun, carving out our own curls of lino from grey blocks, ready to reveal their secrets in the printing studio the next day. My oldest daughter carved the story of my friend Siri the diver, in a portrait of a free-floating diver, hair flowing behind her, in front of the giant eye of a whale.

I climbed the hill with the kids and we looked out as far as the shadowy zigzags of the Lofoten Islands, grey on the far horizon. The water was the deepest blue all the way there, but traces of paler blue snaked around the islands closer in, telling stories of passing boats and sandy patches, the shaping of underwater contours. The nearest mountain, three islands away, was cut off halfway up by cloud.

On the way down, I held my youngest daughter's hand and she started talking to me about her birthday. The thoughts moved on to my grandma, who shared a birthday with her, and her fingers. 'Why are they so wrinkled if she hasn't been in water?' Ellie asked. It was true that her skin was as wrinkled as Ellie's after an hour in the swimming pool, but I told her it was just because she was old, because she had lived a life and it shows in your skin. I remembered that this grandma didn't know how to swim, even though she took us to the beach to collect shells and lark about on lilos for days on end, standing at the water's edge in her short green wellies to watch. The other granny was the champion swimmer. A swimmer and a non-swimmer. Dark and light.

Our return to the dusk-laden streets of Copenhagen was like a re-entry from the moon. Though the days were still warm and long, there was a cold current near the ground. The season's change was well on its way. It was only August but winter was in the post. I was thinking about that big swim ahead in the Stockholm archipelago and whether my nerve would hold as the water cooled. Would I be a strong-minded champion swimmer like one granny, or softer and not so much of an athlete like the other? A week without training – dipping and splashing about by the island was no substitute for laps – had taken that goal a little further away from me, but I was, as always, up for the challenge. I didn't have long to find out if it was a challenge fit for me or not.

22

August in Denmark is the start of a new page in an exercise book, even though it is still the height of summer in the UK. In Denmark, August, not September, is the start of the new school year. I passed a woman putting her towel on the deck on the way to walk my daughter to school, clad in a black swimming costume with white piping, preparing to jump into the canal on the corner where the harbour bus passes. I felt a twinge – I was in a suit jacket and dress, ready for a meeting in town, and my hair was ironed flat. I'd have preferred to be make-up free and in a swimsuit like her.

I hadn't swum properly since we came back from Norway a few weeks ago, though. Something happens in summer: time becomes elastic and routines no longer hold. Days go by without me really thinking about it. I was, probably, swimming every couple of days but the training felt like an idea that belonged to the distant past, to last year, even. The couple of dips I took to cool off on a hot day and humid evening didn't really count: since my swimming-induced earache had disappeared, a pernicious cold had taken its place and I felt like I'd spent weeks sleeping on the sofa, coughing up green bilge instead of sleeping soundly. I read a shocked-sounding report from the UK* that said that around 50 per cent of women have dropped out of doing exercise. Never mind that the report was commissioned by one of the UK's largest sportswear brands (what could possibly be in it for them?), I could understand completely why that would be the case. It doesn't take much for exercise to fall off the priority list. It was always about time.

I loved the time I spent swimming. I loved to swim meditative laps, slow and leisurely, focused on stroke and form. I loved to do interval training, two fast laps and one recovery. I loved to practise diving, pointing my toes, spotting where I wanted to enter the water and sliding in. But with the kids home all summer, limited plans in the air and a stillness coming over the usually ticking clock, all plans seemed to be off. All energy had dissipated. There was no forward movement anymore. My illness had completely made me lose my rhythm and I couldn't find the energy in my bones to get back on the horse and try again. My training scheme for the Stockholm island trip had gone to the dogs.

Since it was the back-to-school month, and time to turn the page, I decided that I needed to shake

* Asics, 'Closing the Gender Exercise Gap': https://www.asics.com/gb/en-gb/mk/move-her-mind

things up again. I needed one night a week to swim. One night to myself. That was all. Since the harbour bath was going to be open for another four weeks, and the jellyfish had all gone on vacation, I decided to head there after the kids were back from school and get back on the open-water swim schedule I'd found online a few weeks ago. First up: swim 700 metres. It was just 28 lengths of the pool.

As 5pm came and went, I wondered if I'd summon up the energy to slip into my swimsuit. I booked a rental car from the street and started walking over the bridge with my swimming bag slung over my arm, thinking about the three saunas and hot pool at the local leisure centre, and the long lanes I'd swim laps in. But then I stopped. There, to the right of me, was the almost empty harbour. The sun was low in the sky, shining right into the harbour pool. I cancelled the car and walked right to it.

The pool was empty apart from three noisy French children who were daring each other to jump in from the platform, and one lady with the elaborate coiled hair of a Russian ballerina. She floated around the pool as I started to sweat out the frustrations of my day, which had been, in no particular order, the dog behaving badly on a walk, a slight anxiety that I didn't have much work booked in beyond Friday, and a general lack of direction. I kept trying to tell myself that it was part of the plan, part of the fallowness of it all that I had lots of space in my diary, but all this space also told a story of being unwanted, unnecessary, surplus to requirements – and I didn't like it.

The first few lengths brought up goosebumps on my skin as I adjusted to the radical change in temperature. It was 17°C in the water, and around 20°C in the air. I felt chilled, but after a few lengths, I stopped noticing the temperature and started noticing the water. I looked at how it dimpled, at how dark and unknowable it was, with the sun at this low angle in the sky. How reflective it was, like a mirror, in the places where we weren't swimming. I felt for the eddies and underwater currents that were herding the long pieces of floating seagrass together in a corner. It was too dark to see if there were jellyfish in the water, but nobody was making a fuss about them, especially not the noisy kids, so I mentally crossed my fingers and carried on. I could feel a little tightness, a stinging around my wrist, as if it had been wrapped with a piece of that long, thin, floating sea grass, but when I looked, there was nothing there. It felt, for the next few hours, like a memory of chilli on my tongue, or the imagining of a burn, but there was nothing to see.

Twenty-eight lengths later and I was out, wrapped in a shabby blue towel, with my Birkenstocks on, walking back home. I thought about something I had read on Twitter about water. It said that the water in your body was just visiting; it will come and go like morning dew. It was beautiful, especially for Twitter. I was full of water, like we all are. I'm refreshed by water as it passes through on to its next place, up to the clouds and down to another river. Maybe it will fall as snow on the glaciers of Greenland, or on the peaks of the Norwegian mountains where the snow sits all year round. Maybe it will fall as rain on the dark, dirty backstreets of Manchester where I used to walk, or on the coiffed hair of a bride on her wedding day. Maybe it will drench an unprepared person on the way to work, or maybe it will lightly spritz the air, turning hair frizzy and beading up on windows. Or it will fall on a dry and cracked garden gasping to be soaked down to the roots so the roses can hold their heads up high and bloom again.

I wonder about the journey the water in my body has been on. Did it once rush the white rapids of a Himalayan river? Have I ever drunk it before? Was it in our harbour, centuries ago, when the ships plied it and mechanical noises drowned out voices, or was it leaping from a carved fountain in a stately home as an object of wonder and delight? Maybe my body's water had once been rippling in a mountain stream in Scotland or caught in a salty rock pool as the tide went out, gradually evaporating in the heat to leave dehydrated fronds of dark seaweed and reclusive limpets, able to wait until the next tide came in. Has it been in you? And her? And them? Has it been a coolant in an engine system or flowed through the pipes of a dishwasher on its way to me? Or has it always been pure, an ancient, unlocked piece of deep iceberg melted by the sun, cracking as it releases its long-held breath of oxygen back to the air and its frozen water back to the sea?

It feels like the closest thing to time travel that I can imagine – a part of me going forward into the future, into another world. It's also a kind of rebirth, a reincarnation: part of me becoming part of a slug, or an eagle, or a whale. It's awesome, in the true sense of the world, when you come to think about it. It's not my water, it's our water. And all is water.

Mid-August, it was blindingly hot outside all day and almost all night. By hot, I mean 27°C in the day, 20°C at night; remember, this is Copenhagen. But it was a particular type of hot, hotter, my Italian friend says, than in Spain and Italy. It was hot right here in our neighbourhood, because the water reflects the heat and then it reflects again against the tall many-windowed apartments, and then it bounces off brickwork and concrete and makes the streets in full sun feel like some kind of furnace. Nobody put any thought into cooling the streets or creating shadowy, narrow walkways or air conditioning because most of the year, heat conservation is much more important.

We were living through a summer heatwave in Europe and, so the news told us, this was just the start of things to come. Even though I knew it was hot and I was glad to have somewhere to cool off just steps away, the thought of autumn still dogged my thoughts, with its darker nights and its unshakable cold.

We swam as a family after school. My older daughter used the swimming pool as a playground with her friends. People clustered around the water, swimming in it, sunbathing next to it, drinking iced coffees all along it. But mid-month, COVID finally tracked me down and I was left watching through the window from my sweat-drenched bed, as everyone else had all the fun. The hope of my swim in Stockholm, around Mags's island, was off for this year. There was just not enough time left in the summer to fit it in. As I rounded six days of suffering, I focused all my energy on being able to dip in the water the next day so I didn't break my swimming streak.

I was also reading about Greenland. Over the past three months, I had gathered up every book about Greenland written in English and stored in the central Copenhagen library system. It was a curious combination of ideas, a motley mixture of books including one about an African who travelled to Greenland in the 1980s, another by an American travel writer who lived and hunted with Inuit, and one by an American Pulitzer Prize winning journalist who focused on the ice and the scientists studying it. In the heat of my bedroom, I imagined what it might be like in September to leave a simple hotel early in the morning and walk to the nearest beach and slip into the water for a swim. I didn't think it would be clean. I anticipated oily water with a residue from fishing boats at the very least. My overture to Nuuk's swimming association had so far drawn a blank: I wrote to a few people on Facebook, but it seemed that people didn't really swim in the open water in Nuuk, apart from one hardy ultra-swimmer, who intimidated me so much I don't follow up. My quest wasn't about adrenaline and achievement, after all. At least not in that way. It was more of a spiritual quest, an internal adventure.

Dawn broke on Sunday and I woke up feeling able to leave my bed again. COVID, for now, was beaten. My husband asked me if I wanted to swim with him before the kids got up, and we swam long, slow strokes from the floating dock in Teglholm across to the orange ladder beside the houseboats on Sluseholmen, and then back again before the kids woke up.

As September approached, the air was cut through with an undercurrent of cold in the mornings, enough for a jumper or jacket, not quite enough for a coat. On an early morning dog walk, though the leaves on the trees were still a silvery green, I saw an orange-brown maple leaf the size of my hand drifting in the canal. I packed my kit for Greenland weeks before I needed to, testing its weight, wondering if my thick parka was too heavy, too warm, or just right. The parka itself was thicker than a duvet and so big. Predicted temperatures for September in Iceland: 15°C. I'd spend a day and a night there, in my beloved Reykjavik, before taking a further five-hour flight to Greenland, where the temperature would drop to just 3.5°C. I couldn't remember what 3.5°C felt like, but I knew I didn't like it. The hot summer had messed with my memories. I forget every year about winter and the dark and what's coming. I tried to get prepared, with multiple pairs of sweat-wicking socks, merino wool underwear and a new woolly hat, but it felt ridiculous in the heat of late summer.

I arranged to swim with Kristín in Iceland, and I finally located a winter swimmers' club in Greenland, via Facebook, who swam every Sunday at 9.30am. They invited me to join them. 'Just show up,' their organiser said, 'but know that there's nowhere to get changed, we just get changed on the beach.' I looked it up on the map, and found it was a small beach in the colonial harbour in the oldest part of Nuuk, a little walk from where I thought I was going to be staying. It felt exciting: I could imagine myself getting up early to go down there before my day's work activities began. Afterwards they would go for coffee to warm up. It sounded perfect.

The week that September broke, I had an extraordinary day. The sun was shining and there was a cold catch in the air, but it was the kind of day that I wanted to grab with both hands and never let go of. I swam slowly from my island to the next and paused by the bright orange ladder to watch the swifts (or swallows, I never know which) dive and swoop for insects on the surface of the water, beside the houseboats and reconditioned ferries.

I swam back, slowly again, sculling on my back, with a view of the pure blue sky.

Later in the morning, I took Max for a walk up the green hill nearby. I let him off the lead and instead of zooming off, like usual, he wandered over to a shady bush and flopped down next to it, panting, out of the sun. It was a sign that summer wasn't over yet.

At the bottom of the hill, we sat in the shade of my favourite café and I treated myself to a croissant. A moment of great happiness, a wave, broke over me, giving me a sense that this was what life was about. I was breathing normally. I could see sunshine playing on water. Max was sitting right beside me with a grin on his face. My family was healthy again, for now, and happy again. I had a head full of ideas and future plans. Everything was golden in the bright sunlight. I was enjoying the little things, and it felt good. We all get to decide what we think a good life is. For now, with the space to reflect, I thought that I had found mine.

23

To say that my year had been building up to my Iceland-Greenland trip was an understatement: I think perhaps my life had been leading up to this one point. In a feat of enormous serendipity, I had managed to arrange the seemingly impossible: a work trip that took in some of the most interesting things I had ever done, with some of the most exciting people possible, in the most extreme environment I had ever been. And there was even time and space for swimming along the way. I had only started winter bathing in Copenhagen ten or so months ago and now I was about to swim at the top of the world, in the coldest seas imaginable.

I kept telling myself: *How cold could it be?* If the water was not frozen, I wasn't being as brave as Leena in Finland, cutting a hole in the ice. I would simply be dipping, just like I have in Copenhagen, just like I have in the Arctic Circle. No big deal. Though as I left for the airport, I spied a report in a Greenlandic newspaper saying that there was a dead whale carcass floating in the water just off Nuuk right now, which added a new frisson to it all.

Part of my mission in Greenland was to write a story exploring the relationship between Greenlanders and nature, and how access to their extraordinary, extreme nature affects their mental health. It was a story I pitched and developed with my editor back in March, when I really only had a rudimentary idea about how the story might unfold. That is normal when I pitch features to editors – I tend to have a rough outline, gleaned from some light research, and go on to develop them in greater detail when I get a thumbs up from them to pursue them. But this one had taken me in a new direction, not quite in the way I'd imagined.

With extra time on the subject, thanks to the delayed trip, I'd had the chance to read books as thick as a step on the subject of Greenlandic culture, Greenlandic explorers and the Greenland ice sheet, and, let's not forget, I've been swimming in the cold Nordic waters of Denmark, Norway and Finland, understanding the link between nature and mental health first hand. It was self-evident to me that being out in nature helps your mental health. It's proven everywhere you look. It was also clear to me that taking people out of their natural rhythms and routines and putting them in offices can be terrible for mental health. Just look at me – and I don't even live in a place as extremely influenced by nature as the Greenlanders.

I spoke to researcher Dr Naja Carina Steenholdt about it before I left. She has spent several years investigating wellbeing in Greenland for her PhD at the University of Aalborg and gleaned some fascinating results.

It all started as a result of a curious paradox that she discovered when researching her Bachelor's and Master's degrees in Copenhagen.

'Research shows that Greenlanders are very happy with their lives,' she said, 'with results overwhelmingly showing very high levels of satisfaction. But our statistics show high suicide rates, big social problems and range of statistics from a Western perspective that do not fit with the idea of people being very happy. With higher than average levels of violence and crime, how can this be a good life? The big question is: what makes a good life?'

With her research team, she started to ask Greenlanders about what they believed to be the foundation for a good life. And they came back with two conclusions: family and social relationships, and nature.

After speaking to over 70 people for her research, she narrowed it down even further. If you were to say one thing that is the secret to a good life in Greenland, it's nature.

'We looked at how important different aspects of life are: family, work, culture, sport and local community included,' she said. 'It really struck me how many people rated nature higher than family. It is not just seen as a source of food – most people in Greenland hunt or fish – it is so fundamental that it overrules family and work. It is the precondition for a good life.

'People would answer: "Without nature, I would have no family. I wouldn't be able to live my life." "I get food and energy from nature." This was a regular response. There is a deep understanding that nature comes before everything. It's a modest, elementary approach to life.'

Dr Steenholdt was curious about how to apply nature to problems that the current health system in the country was at a loss to deal with.

'Most days, nature gives, no matter how you look at it, and makes the negative feel more positive. It's plain and simple,' she said. 'Nature has this powerful feature that it can turn a negative to a positive, so why don't we use it collectively?'

How does nature affect your mental health? How can wild swimming at the top of the world affect your approach to life? How can we all find a way to put a bit of nature and adventure into our lives? These are the questions I found myself asking of myself and of others.

I flew into Reykjavik on an overcast Monday morning and killed time walking the city's back-streets. I realised on my way out there that I had been visiting Reykjavik for almost twenty years – I wrote a guidebook to the city in 2003 – and it was a bittersweet experience to walk the city streets and see how much things had changed. If you've ever returned to your hometown after a long absence, you'll know the feeling: the shops that are no longer there, the nightclubs that have changed name but are still known, among your generation anyway, by their old name. Memories cling to certain streets. I wandered down a street parallel to the main drag amid tumbledown, colourful corrugated-iron houses and the occasional cat peering out from a graffitied driveway. It had crossed my mind ten years ago to buy a flat in the city, and I wholeheartedly regretted that I hadn't taken it further.

I felt a great surge of love for Reykjavik, for its off-beat atmosphere and coloured houses. I loved that the mainly pedestrianised main street had been painted in places so it looked like a racetrack, or a giant game of snakes and ladders, or an Insta-ready rainbow. It was playful. But I hated the fact that every second shop on the street was aimed at tourists. There was a shop full of plastic Viking stuff, another full of expensive Icelandic herbs and delicacies, packed to make the perfect gift. I wondered where the locals went shopping now. I barely heard that lovely Icelandic accent in the air.

I met Kristín at 3.30pm at the white parliament building in the centre of town. It was the Prime Minister's office, and it was both humble and special at the same time. Kristín took me on a little tour, including a peek inside the actual office where the Prime Minister sits – incongruously, she's a Liverpool supporter with an Anfield sign on the wall near her desk, amid some eclectic modern art – before we headed upstairs to meet her colleague Páll, who was coming too. The three of us piled into Kristín's car and picked up her daughter, Sigrún, for a real treat. They were taking me to Hvammsvík natural hot springs, just under an hour out of the city, in a place called Hvalfjordur, the 'whale fjord'.

Hvammsvík had only been opened for a few months and was one of at least three natural and geothermally heated spas to have opened in the last year in Iceland. That's on top of the famed Blue Lagoon, and Vök, Mývatn Nature Baths and Geosea, all thermal spas that have been around for a while. The difference between this one and many of the others is that it was right on the bay, not perched on a cliff with views of the sea. It was made up of seven rounded hot tubs enclosed by great boulders, steaming gently in the cooling afternoon air, and one tidal pool, gradually being erased by the incoming tide. All this, and it was overlooked by sheer moss-covered mountains, with dark grey scree falling down the sides and scars where glaciers once raked their sides. The sky was heavy with light grey clouds. We changed in a former barracks building dating back to the Second World War. On the wall as we went in there was a display of photos of Land Rovers stuck in Iceland's rivers, water rising to cover the tyres. The drivers had overestimated their abilities in the face of the challenge. It was a little note about Icelandic nature: it is definitely stronger than anything you can imagine, and is always ready to outwit you.

Out in the bay, there were two grass-tufted islands, and from the corner of my eye, I thought I saw a seal. On second glance, it was not a seal at all but the oily back of a large cormorant, diving for a fish. On the way, I asked the Icelanders if there were still whales in the whale fjord but they said probably not. In a cruel twist of irony, the few whales still hunted 'for scientific purposes' in Iceland were brought to and processed on this very fjord.

As there often is in Iceland, a folk story underpins the name of the fjord. An elf woman, angered at her human lover's refusal to recognise their child, transformed him into an angry red-headed whale as revenge. The whale, so the story goes, lived in the fjord, wrecking ships for years to come.

Páll was already swimming in the sea when we stepped out from the changing room, and we rushed out to join him. Well, I should say that they rushed out. The air temperature was around 10°C, the water around 8°C. It had been a while since I'd swum in water this cold. The numbers seemed fine in theory – after all, I'd swum in much colder water – but as I stumbled through ankle-deep water across the dark pebbles and nuggets of pumice stone, I got a life lesson. It was really cold. I struck out to join the Icelanders, who were swimming with gloves and swim socks on, but otherwise just swimsuits, and I could only get halfway before I just couldn't go any further. My feet iced up. It was like that day swimming with Mette under her flat all over again. I just couldn't do it.

It was not surprising at all: Hvalfjörður is deep and 30 kilometres long, connecting to the North Atlantic Ocean. There is an undersea tunnel passing underneath it that slopes steeply to the deepest point, 165 metres below the surface, that I've driven a couple of times and always felt spooked by. There's just so much water above you, and the drive is uncommonly steep. I swam back to the shore and clambered over the rocks into the semi-submerged tidal hot pool to warm up my chilly bones.

I felt like a terrible fraud. To myself and to them. On the way there in the car, I had talked about how I was going to swim in Greenland. But I couldn't even swim here, in this water. I had been fooling myself just a bit. I told myself that these Icelanders swam much more regularly in cold water than I did, and after all, the warm water of Copenhagen this summer had spoilt me. Maybe they had more ice in their blood, by nature of genetics – like Icelandic fisherman Guðlaugur Friðþórsson in Bonnie Tsui's *Why We Swim*, perhaps they share an extraordinary genetically-born resilience to the cold. Maybe they're just a lot tougher than me. I recalibrated in the tidal pool, which was now half warm water and half cold fjord water, and watched Kristín, Sigrún and Pall floating about on their backs, black-socked feet sticking up like flippers, with great big smiles on their faces like they were in a heated pool in the Med.

I swam halfway out to them again as they swam back in, sad I couldn't tolerate the cold enough to join them, but happy to be with them anyway. Kristín fished out a small blue-veined jellyfish with her neoprene gloves, and held it in her hand before gently moving it out of the way. I was surprised the water was warm enough for them. None of us had ever been stung.

I asked Sigrún what the Icelandic word for jellyfish was. '*Marglyttur*,' she said. 'It means ... sea glitter, I think.' I told them that the Danish word was '*vandmand*' – water man. It was funny that Icelandic is so wantonly poetic, as full of magic as an incantation, where Danish is just straightforward, say what you see. She said that she'd read some Israeli research* about jellyfish, stating that they are affected by the full moon, and in the days before and during it, they come into the shore in swarms. There was a full moon a few nights ago; I remembered it hanging low and huge over the streets of Copenhagen.

The seawater pools were delightfully half empty on this Monday late afternoon, and the people who were there were chatty. I talked to a man who lived close by, in Mosfellsbær, and to an English-Canadian woman who worked with horses nearby. She was shocked that we were all swimming in the sea, and we told her she should try it. I held her phone and videoed her going in for the first time. When she came out, she couldn't stop talking about how warm she felt. She looked lit up. Honestly, converting someone to a cold-water dip is like being a vampire and turning someone to the dark side. You know once

* https://phys.org/news/2016-08-moon-key-jellyfish-beach.html#:~:text=In%20the%20middle%20of%20the,stinging%20humans%2C%20the%20research%20found.

they've tried it, they will want to do it again, and it feels good to induct them into something so niche.

Before we left, I tried to swim in the fjord again. I got thigh-deep and duck-dived under. My feet were still crying out in pain and I couldn't stay in for long, but at least there was that. It's not a competitive experience, swimming in cold water, but I still felt like I'd let myself down, that I had failed somehow. It was a reminder again that even when I thought I'd cracked it, I still had a long way to go, clearly, in my cold-water tolerance and in my integration into Nordic life. It seemed like one equalled the other. But on the way back to the city in the car, I was reminded that this wasn't a Viking test of strength, and that there was something more valuable to gain from all of this than staying in cold water until your toes froze right off.

We sped back to Reykjavik and listened to Páll's tales of dating life in the city, and chatting about where Damon Albarn lived, here on the northern outskirts, with a perfect view of the sea. The swimming was fun and the spa was fun, but you know what? This was the best. We laughed and talked all the way back to the city. It was mad to think that swimming brought me here, all the way from the fifteen-degree water of Copenhagen harbour and into a community that was this fun to belong to.

24

After talking to Dr Steenholdt about Greenlanders and their relationship with nature, I started thinking about how nature and living a good life intersect even more. I wondered if nature had to be big, painted on a huge canvas, to do you good, or whether just the sight of trees in a city and the odd rose bush in a park could do the same thing. Should it be awesome, or could it be more mundane? It was clear from the off that nature in Greenland was the main character in everyone's lives, and perhaps that's what makes the biggest difference.

It took an hour to reach Uunartoq by boat, an island in a fjord lined with dark and jagged kilometre-high mountains, ancient volcanoes with their tops blown off. This part of south Greenland is volcanic, and one of the very few places in the country with a natural hot spring.

On the way to it, the skipper said that a few years ago he had accidentally driven into a surfacing whale in this exact place, and been flung from the boat into ice-cold water. He was lucky to survive. The fjord was remote, unpopulated in recent times, though it had a small hamlet a generation ago that was forcibly moved into a larger settlement. As we passed by it, the four wooden houses stood eerily empty, with dark windows like a mouth full of broken teeth, looking at us as we went by. There was no doubting that the beautiful turquoise water was cold: as we closed in on the island, four icebergs the size of a three-storey house casually drifted by. After the whale collision, the skipper and his boatmates made it back to the boat and carried on, though one of them had a bloody nose, having hit his head on the steering wheel as he collided with the whale. The whale itself was fine, he said.

It was a short walk up a scrubby hillside to the hot springs. After swimming in Iceland, and finding the cold almost completely unbearable, this was exactly what I needed. I sank into the 37°C water and dug my toes into the hot, dark sand, trying to find an even warmer spot. The air temperature was a cool 11°C. Bubbles came up in a long line from under the silty bottom of the pool, making it feel like a gentle jacuzzi, and as the wind got up, I looked past the boulders to see the icebergs drifting along the fjord. If there was a better view to be had from any hot tub or hot spring anywhere in the world, I'd like to know about it.

This little hot spring had played host to some very hardy people in days gone by: at this very hot spot, the Greenlandic Vikings rested their aching muscles a thousand years ago. They enlarged the pool that local Inuit were already using and moved the larger boulders that encircle it today. I had a moment sitting in it, alongside my group which included a strapping Icelander and a tattooed and bearded Dane, thinking about what it must have looked like a thousand years ago, who was wallowing here, and what sort of tattoos they might have had.

I don't think the views would have been tremendously different; the boats hitched to the dock would have been replaced by small wooden boats pulled up to the beach, and the path up here may have been shorter and steeper as a result, but the mountains, the iceberg views and the fjord would have been the same. Given the access the Vikings had to hot water (i.e. none) and the amount of sheep farming, walrus hunting and polar bear wrangling they must have been doing, I'm not sure the water would have been so clean, though.

I wallowed in this lovely bath for half an hour before I forced myself to get out and put on my long johns and coat, over the top of my swimsuit. Then I walked down a hillside dotted with crowberry shrubs and rocks to a protected curve of white sand beach backed with gentle dunes. There was not a footprint in sight. Perfectly clear and calm turquoise water lapped the sand, decorated with mussel shells and light drifts of kelp. If I didn't know better, it could have been Caribbean water, and if it had been, this pretty beach would have made the world's best beaches lists for sure. The four huge icebergs were now floating in the water about 200 metres away. I stripped off my long johns, leaving them in a pile with my coat, walked to the water's edge and went straight in. I duck-dived under when the water hit my upper thighs and swam. It took my breath away.

I swam until my skin was burning and I started to lose the feeling in my fingers. It did not take long.

Then I ran up and down the beach to warm myself up before I went back in to swim again. My feet sank ankle deep into the loosely compacted sand, and I made a real mess of this perfect beach with my footprints, but it was worth it. Back in the water again, this time for longer, I got that wonderful all-body glow that lit me up inside. As I walked out of the water, my skin the pinkish-red of a freshly boiled lobster, I felt full of an electric energy, fearless, fuelled by that pep of adrenaline you can only get from cold-water swimming.

I wrapped myself in my towel, put on my coat and ran up the hill in the now freezing wind and threw myself back into the warmth of the hot spring. It only took a minute or two to warm up, and then I began to wish I had stayed down by the invigorating Arctic Sea. It nixed all those feelings of not being good enough that I'd had in Iceland. None of that mattered: I felt like an adventurer, for just a handful of seconds. The Reykjavik fjord had been full of energy and history too, but this one, with its clear sea, the fine sand beach and the admittedly rather ramshackle changing-room setup, felt pure. My eyes briefly clouded with happy tears: an upwelling of emotion at being a tiny person alive in such a huge landscape.

On the return boat trip, a small Minke whale briefly surfaced in the fjord, a semi-circle of back fleetingly curving out of blue to remind me that swimming here was usually just for the wild things. It felt good for a moment or two to be one of them.

As the days went on, I felt completely blown away by Greenland. My senses were overstimulated from dawn till dusk. I sat in a boat, watching icebergs with eyes full of wonder. When opaque grey sea mist gathered and thickened around the boat, my head swirled with memories of the books I had been reading in the summer. I saw the ghosts of the latter-day adventurers in my mind, the men who arrived on the shore of this unknown land and found pack ice that encroached on their boats and held them so tight that the oak timbers groaned and eventually splintered. This unknown land looked unknowable to me; every chunk of ice that pinged off the bottom of our metal boat made me jump, and the sound of our vessel cutting through the water, thick and granulated with ice like a slushie, felt full of foreboding. Having a vivid imagination in a place like this seemed like a blessing and a curse: a curse because it makes you think of all the many terrifying ways you can die and the incredibly hostile creatures out there, each one growing hungrier as the winter comes round and the darkness falls. But a blessing because at least you'd be able to entertain people with stories in those dark winter months when you need something to pass the time.

There's a long tradition of storytelling linked with nature in Greenland, and a long list of terrifying mythical beasts as a result. Imagine: a magical polar bear as tall as a mountain who sucks up kayakers with his nostrils. A half-human, half-animal mountain dweller who likes to dissemble and attack anyone who sneaks up onto its hillside uninvited. And then there's the Mother of the Sea. She's my favourite, for a number of reasons.

The Mother of the Sea was once a human, and according to one version of the legend, she was in a kayak hunting with her family when a storm started. Her father thought she was to blame for the storm, and threw her in the sea. As she reached up and clung to the kayak, he cut off her fingers, first the tips, then the second knuckle and then the last knuckle. She sank down to the very bottom of the sea.

There, at the bottom of the Greenlandic Sea, she lives in a little peat house guarded by a giant dog, and acts as the mother, creator and protector of all the creatures living beneath the sea. It's an important job. When humans are selfish, pollute the sea, overfish it or break her many taboos, she gathers up all the animals of the sea and hides them in her long dark hair, leading to famines and poor fishing for the people of Greenland. The only way to solve the issue is to send the local shaman down to comb her hair. Then she, the spirit of the sea, releases the creatures back to the surface via a freshwater stream that runs from the doorway of her house.

It's a well-loved and well-known story about environmental protection central to a culture from way before we were talking about it in the Western world. In a country where the sea is a deep larder that everyone eats from, it's a story about behaving well, looking after each other, and seeing it as a person who also deserves respect. At the time I researched the Mother of the Sea, a company in the UK had just put 'nature' on their board of directors, keen to give it a vote on any major corporate issue, and the CEO of Patagonia decided to donate all the company's profits to fight climate change. They both seemed like significant, landmark decisions about how nature should be at the heart of all our decision making; in Greenland, that's the way it's always been.

There was a statue of the Mother of the Sea at the spot where Nuuk's winter bathing club met every Sunday at 9am. Bare breasted and powerful, she holds a polar bear, walrus and countless seals close to her as she stares out from a spot on a big broad rock that is uncovered at low tide, but which places her floating in the sea as it comes in. That was not why they met here, or at least it was not the only reason. There was a small patch of sand near the larger slabs of rocks, and it was a central place in the old colonial harbour, near the Greenland Museum and a church on a hill which chimes nine times: local swimmers gird their loins on a Sunday to plunge into the cold water on the ninth tone.

But I wasn't there on a Sunday to meet the local swimming people as arranged. The unpredictable weather in Greenland threw me off course and I found myself in a large town called Qaqortoq for a few more days than I had expected, instead of on the beach with them. Nature was in charge above all things, and you couldn't fight it.

As the winds and waves proved too high to explore the nearby fjords, islands and towns as planned, I sloped off to a lake at the back of the town for the afternoon, where the day before I'd seen some kids swimming. I was intrigued. There wasn't a swimming pool in Qaqortoq – in fact, there were only a handful in Greenland overall. Nuuk got its first swimming pool in 2003, a beautiful wave-shaped pool with floor-to-ceiling windows, close to the pond where people used to learn to swim, but for a fishing, boat-bound nation, swimming was a surprisingly low-priority activity.

Tasersuaq, Qaqortoq's lake, as the town's main water supply, was filled with fresh water, with rocky islands poking up at various points within it, and a flat hiking trail circling it, the foothills of mountains extending behind it. The mountains were bare, with browning autumn grass and hardy shrubs of thyme and crowberry all over them.

At a gathering spot behind a series of what looked like red municipal housing blocks, six children were playing at the water's edge. Two boys clad in wet-suits hauled themselves out of the water, climbed to the highest rocks and threw themselves off, trying to get as far into the water as they could. Another boy was swimming in the water with a big snorkel mask, looking under the water. A little dumpling of a girl who must have been about eight was standing on the edge in a woolly jumper and houndstooth trousers, while two others larked about on the shore beside a bike.

I asked them, in tentative Danish, if I could swim there too, and if this was the best spot for swimming around the lake. They mostly ignored me, but the boy closest to me said, 'Yes, it's here or the beach on the other side of town.' I got changed quickly and hopped in, meaning to swim to a group of rocks about a hundred metres away and then back. But I got that same cold shock I had in Iceland and only made it about halfway before realising that even if I could get there without my fingers freezing, I wouldn't be able to make it back. The boys carried on flinging themselves off the rocks.

I swam back, then climbed up the rocks and dived in. The cold made my head shiver, but it felt good.

I made it to Nuuk on an overcast day when the mountains, horizon and anything else that might be considered scenic, interesting or inspiring were hidden by a big drift of grey clouds. I immediately wrote it off as the most depressing place I'd ever been.

A few days before, I had written a call-out to anyone in the Nuuk winter swimming club to see if anyone would swim with me on another day, not a

Sunday, as I knew I had missed their regular session. Nobody had replied.

So I carried on with the work I was there to do, interviewing local experts and attending meetings and press conferences. At one, I met Merete, an editor at the Greenlandic national newspaper, and she was kind enough to say she'd meet me for lunch. Over *smørrebrød* in Nuuk's smartest business hotel, we chatted about life in Greenland. She gave me the chance to ask all the questions I wanted to ask: How has she noticed the effects of climate change in her daily life? Has she ever seen a polar bear? And could she help me with my side quest: a mission to swim in the sea one last time while I was in Nuuk?

Merete, who knew everyone in Nuuk, was able to find me a local winter bather, of course. She texted me later to say that Michael would meet me and take me swimming.

Michael was in his fifties, a former politician and businessman who had a little time to spare today after helping his granddaughter with her homework. I counted myself lucky to have him on hand to answer all my questions about swimming in Greenland: How many people are there in his club? Does he like it, really, even in the depths of winter? Why did he start swimming in the first place? None of the answers he gave me were the ones I was expecting, not least his reason for swimming to begin with. It was, he said, down to the bees.

According to Michael, there's a thing about Greenlanders and bees. 'If you look up Greenlandic memes, you'll find it pretty quickly,' he said. Apparently, these resourceful people who survive and thrive on this beautiful but inhospitable island where every single town records below zero temperatures through the winter are scared of bees. Not mosquitoes, of which there are so many in summer it's impossible to count them. Not polar bears, which are rare in some parts of the country and so abundant in others that hikers have to take rifles with them on a walk. Not any number of wild animals, in fact, from whales, to orca, to walrus, to narwhals. But bees.

Michael told me that he was really afraid of bees. But then he got stung by one, when he was a student in the Pacific Northwest. It wasn't that bad. It wasn't anything like he had expected, and it made him think a little about the nature of fear and how it had stopped him from doing things he might otherwise have done. And how fear might be misplaced, and you could live all your life not doing things, even though they weren't as bad as you imagined, if you let it control you.

Soon after that, he faced another fear: swimming in the sea. The opportunity came up in May, a month designated for doing healthy activities in Greenland. He went for it and surprised himself. Even so, he confessed, every time is a challenge. If he wasn't part of the winter swimming group, he thought he wouldn't do it. It was always hard. I could definitely empathise. His absolute favourite thing was the hot shower he took at home after a swim, and the restful, relaxed feeling he had after that. Today, I had presented him with a challenge, and an opportunity to swim somewhere different: a little beach near the airport that he'd driven past before but never swum at. So he was up for it. And now I had set myself up for it too, and I couldn't back out.

I also had the feeling that he was being modest. After all, he brought me two towels and a pair of socks to protect my feet from the rocks. The man knew what he was doing. We stashed our bags way up the beach because, he told me, sometimes boats came by quickly and brought a bigger than expected wave high up the beach. I started to get my swimming costume out of my bag and he shook his head. In Greenland, apparently, I would be swimming in the nude, just like the Mother of the Sea herself. It was, so it seemed, the smartest way to do it, so there would be less time shivering on the beach in the cold. I'd done it before, I reasoned, so why the hell not.

I stripped off mega quickly and picked my way down the seaweed-stained stones into the shallow water wishing that for once, there would be a big drop just by the shore, not a gently shelving beach that didn't get deep for ages. My feet were icing up before I was able to even get my shoulders under the water, and then I was there, my chest was tight and I was in the water, floating and trying to find my breath. I was swimming naked, apart from socks, in Greenland. I can't say I remember much more of it all very clearly, as the unexpected nudity caused me to disassociate wildly. In fact, I think I might actually have been more scared of being naked in public than I had ever been about swimming in very cold water.

'Is this something you do often?' Michael asked, when he made it into the water too. 'Swimming naked in the sea with strange men?'

He meant it as a joke, but it was true. My behaviour is a bit questionable sometimes.

As I dried myself really quickly and squeezed my still-wet legs into my tight skiing leggings, a powerful inner glow switched on and I felt all bubbly again. 'I miss it, swimming in really cold water like this,' I told him. 'It hasn't felt the same in the warm water in Denmark this summer. I much prefer winter swimming.'

Michael just laughed. 'Winter swimming? In Greenland we do winter swimming all year round. It's just called swimming.'

V. A year of swimming in Scandinavia

25

One morning in early October, we stood at the window and stared at skeins of geese drawing lines across the pale pink early morning sky. Hundreds of birds were leaving Copenhagen on this beautiful clear day on a journey to the warmer climes of Spain and North Africa. As we walked to school, the glorious autumn sun shone with a golden warmth as if it was never going to stop, though the wind carried ice with it on the breeze. For all of us, change was coming.

I took the dog for a walk to a rumoured new swimming spot fifteen minutes across the bridge and along a long straight path that led out to sea. It was the route the seal must have taken when it swam into the harbour late last autumn. The tide was pulling strong chevron shapes and parallel lines in the navy-blue water. I wondered if it was out there in the channel, seeking out the smaller mackerel in the deep water. I hoped he would come into the harbour again this winter.

The new floating platform was positioned, so a big sign said, to allow people to relax in nature. It was a better spot than a bench beside the straight tarmac path here; on weekends, the path was jostling with aggressive male cyclists in Lycra doing time trials, as well as people walking dogs, children in inline skates and Sunday cyclists, rolling two or three abreast. It was not the most relaxing place. Down the bank and by the water, on a lazy Monday morning, the floating platform was like an escape to another world, a trip down a rabbit hole that nobody else could see.

There was a metal ladder at the end of the floating dock leading into the deep blue water. In the shallows I could see a chunky mint green electric bike, the type you could rent by the minute from the street. It was not going anywhere anymore. There was also a little metal sign screwed to the wood of the dock next to the ladder that warned against swimming because of the strong currents. So even though it looked like the perfect swim spot, there was to be no swimming here. I felt disappointed. I so wanted to swim in the deep dark water and to feel its current all around me. It looked so clean and vital.

As my year of swimming was coming to a close, I was thinking about what was next. Twelve months of prioritising the things that made me feel alive above all the other things that I'd always believed I 'had' to put above my own joy had had an incredible effect on my psyche. The person who had climbed tentatively down the metal ladder into the harbour was not the same person as the one who had just swum alone on a beach in Greenland, in a sea full of whales. It was as if every dip in the water had washed away a mask I'd been wearing and I was left, at the end of it all, with myself. I'd followed the things that had made me happy: swimming, meeting new people, and being creative, and it had led me here, back to me, back to who I wanted to be. But what next?

I knew that it wasn't sustainable to carry on this experiment forever, much as I may have wanted to. I needed to take these learnings into a new life, perhaps a more structured one. With the confidence that had come from doing my own thing and seeing it flourish, I now had bigger writing plans and projects to start on. I'd come a long way from living life in service to my inbox and feeling handcuffed to a computer or a meeting room, and I knew I'd never go back to that again, but perhaps there was some way I could work with other people and be part of something bigger than myself too.

I went swimming a couple of times with Hanna and the water was cold but familiar, greenish in the weak sunshine. I dived in from the top of the steps, pushing out deep from the deck, and I ducked my head underwater as I swam back to the steps, but although I was cold and couldn't swim for long, I didn't feel that addictive tingle. At least, not yet. I had to force myself just to go. Maybe I needed it to be colder or maybe I needed something different.

Sosun, who I had swum with at New Year, texted me out of the blue to go kayaking with her on a sunny Saturday morning and I went, without hesitation. I loved it. It was so peaceful and calm to sit in the water and cruise around the canals. When I thanked her for it afterwards, she said she was glad to have someone impulsive she could call when she was feeling impulsive too.

I started thinking about joining a winter swimming club, despite the fact I didn't think I was a club person. I just felt the need for something new.

I invited some friends round for a clothes swap one Sunday and one of them turned out to be an avid winter swimmer. It also turned out she knew a new place where there was a sauna and an ice bath. She was going in a couple of Sundays – so I said I'd join her. Just as I was looking for a different winter swimming group, it seemed to materialise in front of me. This new place had a breathing workshop, an ice bath section and a *saunagus* and, get this, it was even in my part of town. It was open on a Saturday, a day when I was not already committed to a few thousand other things. I booked immediately, pushing the thought of my not very impressive freezing-cold Icelandic swim well out of my mind. Maybe I just needed a bit more practice?

Reflecting on what it has been like to spend a year swimming in cold water in and around Scandinavia, it's been a journey out of my comfort zone, and I feel quite a different person at the end of it. It's a cliché to say that I feel more resilient, but I do. I don't get cold quite as easily as I did before, and I'm not fazed by challenges in quite the same way. I still get daunted, stressed and overwhelmed, but I'm out in the world trying new things, meeting new people and coming up with new projects, which is all a long way away from where I was.

In a small way, I feel like the swimming has helped me rewild myself. By that, I mean sharpen my animal instincts and listen to my body, chase joy and behave in a more animal way. I feel like I've been working on computers for too long, starting at a small screen and missing the bigger picture. I'm a human being alive in the world and I want to grab it with both hands.

One of the topics that has surfaced a lot for me over the year has been: What makes a good life? I've been thinking about it as I've met passionate people around Scandinavia, and as I've travelled and thought about local cultures and landscapes and behaviour. Everywhere I have been, the ingredients to a good life involve nature. The Danish/Norwegian concept of *friluftsliv* is a shorthand for this – it means you should enjoy a life lived in the fresh air, whatever the weather. Now, instead of writing about it in a strip-lit office, I'm out there doing it.

The other component to a good life in these parts of Northern Europe is *hygge* – or *kos*, if you're living in Norway, or *lagom*, in Sweden. All these untranslatable words mean, in one way or another, enjoying the moment, celebrating the small things, not too little, not too much. It's about taking delight in the fabric of life, in living this rich moment, right now. That's not to say that you can linger in the moment for too long – punctuality is a key feature of these countries too, perhaps harking back to a time when if you didn't plan precisely for the months ahead, the snow would come before you were ready. Nature has its distinct seasons and you need to be prepared ahead of time for them. This sense of timing, combined with the idea of celebrating charming moments, is a secret to life in the Nordics.

Another theme has pursued me all year: living intentionally. The way I see it, it's about making decisions about how you want to live and what values you believe in, rather than falling into things because you're expected to, because it's easier to do it, or because everyone else is doing it. I'm in awe of the women and men I've met over the year who fight convention and find their own way to make themselves happy: Siri with her diving and her business; Håvard with his passion for life and creativity; Kristín with her love of the water; Karin, the mermaid who loves undersea life, and so many more.

Every choice you make is a chance to live your values and live a life that feels right for you. Be brave. Choose your own adventure, because this is your life and you're the only one who's going to live it.

It took burnout for me to discover this richer seam to life and I feel so grateful for it. While I can't say I'll never feel down or hopeless again, I do know that nothing makes me feel as happy and alive as swimming in an ice-cold sea. That extraordinary rush of energy is what I need to keep me happy and healthy. I look at the pictures of me exiting the sea in Greenland when I feel a bit hemmed in, just to remind myself of how sparkly I can feel, on a very good day. I hope you find your spark too. I hope you find the energy to get curious and search for it. It might be in the most unlikely of places. Maybe I'll see you in the sea.

FURTHER READING

There are some fantastic books out there about swimming, some of which inspired my writing, and some which provide more depth on the subject. Start with *Waterlog*, Roger Deakin's seminal book about swimming around the UK, and its excellent partner, *The Swimmer*, a biography of Deakin by Patrick Barkham. *Swimming with Seals* by Victoria Whitworth takes on swimming in Orkney and how it helped the author deal with loss. For those keen for a more scientific approach, Wallace J. Nichols's book *Blue Mind* includes deep research on how water makes you happier, more connected and better at what you do. Bonnie Tsui's *Why We Swim* is a great history of the pursuit and includes an intriguing tale of a shipwrecked sailor in Iceland that I enjoyed reading immensely. If you read Icelandic, Kristín Jórunn Hjartardóttir's book *Fær I Flestan Sjó* charts her inspiring Icelandic adventures. David Thomson's *The People of the Sea* is a seminal text on selkies and folklore, the magical elements of swimming in the sea that also add some inspiration to the pursuit. And finally,

Tove Jansson's *Letters from Tove* is a collected set of her letters home after creative adventures around the world; *The Summer Book* is my favourite of all her other books, full of small adventures and the tight focus of island life where you can hear and see the sea everywhere you go.

ACKNOWLEDGEMENTS

This book is dedicated to the memory of Sarah Woodall.

Sarah arranged the trip to Greenland I took in this book, and was instrumental in introducing me to the adventurous country in her role as the Destination Manager of South Greenland. Long after my trip, we shared messages about swimming, swapped photos of the coldest places we'd swum, and planned future swims together. A lover of nature, wilderness and wildness herself, she had supported my growing passion for cold-water swimming and my growing interest in Greenland, which has continued long after this first trip. She passed away unexpectedly while I was editing the final version of this book. I'm enormously sad I can't share it with her, and consider myself incredibly lucky to have met her and shared experiences with her at all. I wish I could swim with her one more time.

I owe a huge thank you to my family. When I first floated the idea of leaving my job with nowhere lined up next, and that I would, vaguely, live off my savings and find a way to make it work, lesser beings would have encouraged me to get real. Not my family. So, thank you to Matt, Olivia and Ellie, for their acceptance that this was something that had to be done, their occasional companionship in the water, and for helping me make it all work. I love you. I hope it will be the springboard to even more adventures and I hope it will help you to find a way to live a life less ordinary and more fulfilling too.

To my dear writer friends, especially Libby Jeffrey, Davina Rungasamy, Gwyneth Rees and Ri Fedosiuk, thank you, thank you, thank you. This book wouldn't have been the same without your help and support. Life is an adventure just having people like you in my life; long may it continue.

Thanks to Julian Alexander, without whose thoughtful encouragement and support this book would not have made it this far. Thanks for your belief in me and in the life-changing power of water. And to Sheryl Garrett: I'm just so happy to have found you as a coach and remain in awe of everything you've ever done. It's great to have you in my life. Now please, go swim in the sea.

Thank you to all the swimmers I interviewed, swam with and quoted in this book. Some names have been changed for privacy, but you know who you are. Thanks to Linn in Bergen; Christina, Sosun, Jette and Hanne, Karin, Effi, Hanna, Sonia and Kasia in Copenhagen; Kristín, Sigrun and Páll in Iceland; Siri, Håvard and Dagmar in Norway; Merete and Michael in Greenland; Leena and Ylva in Finland; and so many other people who have given up their time and swum with me. I hope it won't be the last time.

Thanks to all the tourist boards who have helped me out in my story planning and who have connected me to the unique swimmers they know, and to all the editors who commissioned me for work, not always realising I was doing this side project too. Ilze Pole in particular, a huge thank you to you: your first commission, sending me to Bergen that dark winter, was the thing that kickstarted it all. Ellie Cobb, thank you so much for taking my first pitch on going to the Arctic Hideaway, and for your ongoing support. The adventure it sparked was worth it. Also, Tanny Por, Katinka Friis, Kasper Iversen, Kathrine Lind Gustavsson, Leena Karppinen, Mathilde Rübberdt, Harald Hansen: thank you, thank you, thank you, for all your help and support, for the ideas, the connections and, especially, the logistical planning which, as you know, does not always come as easily to me as it does to you.

A book like this doesn't come together without a brilliant editing team and fantastic publicity support, and the most beautiful cover design ever. Thank you so much to Connor Stait and the team at Icon for everything they have done. What started as a solo attempt has ended up as a team pursuit and it has made it all the better. I'm lucky that this book found you.

Thanks, too, to you, for reading this. It means a lot. I hope it can be the springboard to adventure and a happier life, however you want to do it.